DIET-FREE ME!

HOW TO STOP STRUGGLING LOSE WEIGHT, AND EMBRACE A HEALTHY LIFESTYLE

PAMELA BURKE

Diet-Free Me
How to Stop Struggling, Lose Weight, and Embrace a Healthy Lifestyle

Paperback ISBN: 978-0692782637

Disclaimer

The information in this book is based on my own experience. The information provided herein is for educational and inspirational purposes only. The book does not provide medical advice.

This book is not intended to be a substitute for the medical advice of a licensed physician. The reader should consult with their doctor in any matters relating to his/her health before changing their diet or beginning any exercise regimen, or with any questions they may have regarding a medical condition or treatment.

Do not disregard professional medical advice or delay seeking it, or avoid or delay treatment because of something you have read in this book. Individuals and their bodies vary in innumerable ways. No individual result should be seen as typical.

The author and publisher of *Diet-Free Me* specifically disclaim all responsibility for any liability, loss, or risk, personal or otherwise, incurred as a consequence, directly or indirectly, of the user and/or application of any of the contents of this book.

Editing by Audra Gerber
Book Cover Consultation by Cristina Olds
Book Cover Design by Heidi Sutherlin
Interior Book Design by Heidi Sutherlin and Jen Henderson
Book Illustration by Anandhito Galih Respati

PRAISES FOR *DIET-FREE ME*

WOW! I found *Diet-Free Me* ENGAGING (I talked to myself throughout), quite ENTERTAINING (LOL at times, forgetting where I was) yet, still VERY informative and not preachy. I found quite a bit of myself within the chapters. And as I'm really trying to stay focused and keep on track with my healthy lifestyle, yet AGAIN, I always find my MORTAL enemy to be my eating habits. However, I can DEFINITELY say I will try many of the suggestions throughout *Diet-Free Me* and figure out a way to make them work for me.

Shawnette Goodman, Making life changes while juggling
the joys of being a wife, mother, and full-time worker

I really enjoyed the introduction and the set-up of *Diet-Free Me*. The flexibility of reading beyond Chapter 4 in whatever order is necessary/appropriate or particular interest/priority for the reader is appealing. One of the messages that continues to ring loud in *Diet-Free Me* for me is "Any amount of time you put forth to make time for working out and to take care of your well-being is better than making no time at all." In doing SOMETHING I feel so much better than doing nothing and now celebrate the smallest of achievements.

Davina Brittingham, Being all right with putting myself first in order to be a
healthier me and the best caregiver to my mother and pre-teen daughter

Diet-Free Me is great!!! It's an encouraging, quick, and easy read. In it, Pamela provides her success road map to losing weight and embracing a healthy lifestyle, which gives the reader the tools they need to be successful too! Her road map can also be "tweaked" to your preference.

Kimberly McDoyle, Wife, daughter, lover of my family, and
working professional working to be a better version of me

DIET-FREE ME
FREE COMPANION RESOURCES

pamelaburke.com/dietfreeme-resources

Inside the pages of *Diet-Free Me* are references to bonus resources. The resources include downloadable worksheets, cheat sheets, and other useful content to assist you on your journey to embracing a healthy lifestyle diet-free.

Over time I will continue to add content to this area, therefore be sure to visit the web address below to get your free instant access.

Visit the following link to get free access to your *Diet-Free Me* bonus materials now:

pamelaburke.com/dietfreeme-resources

DEDICATION

To my parents, for working so hard to give
me opportunities you did not have...

To Mom, for instilling in me the passion to help others...

To Kelly, for being the best teammate ever...

And to you, for allowing me to share my
passion for making a positive difference.

CONTENTS

Your struggle is real, but life becomes more fruitful when you fight the good fight and win. Prepare to triumph!

YOU MOST CERTAINLY ARE NOT ALONE

Have you ever looked in the mirror, hating the extra rolls, the droopy stomach, and the thunderous thighs staring back at you? Have you hidden away from friends because of how you let your body go? Has a bigger-sized you made you feel less than confident? Have you lost weight before, only to gain it back—plus some?

That is starting off with a lot of questions, but some people reading this book have experienced at least one, if not all, of those thoughts and feelings. One such person is the one who wrote this book—me.

I imagine that you know what needs to be done in order to feel differently and lose weight. Most people know what they *should* do. We know that it requires exercise and diet. You have probably tried both.

In fact, you may not have much trouble starting an exercise routine. Instead, your Achilles' heel is the diet (the food you eat)—that's the hard part. What do you eat? When do you eat it? How much do you eat? Do you allow yourself a "cheat day"? Giving up your favorite "you know they ain't no dang good for you" foods is a challenge. You have a crazy, unpredictable schedule, which is only made more challenging by the poor options that are readily available. Sometimes you suffer from food cravings, such as thinking that you must have something crunchy yet salty, sugary, or chocolaty.

Then, to combat ALL of that, when you finally decide you are going do what you need to do in order to eat healthier, you read information telling you what you should or should not eat and when you should and should not eat it. Eat low-fat. No, eat high protein. No, do not eat carbs. Do not eat carbs after 5:00—or is it after 6:00? Or is that a bunch of nonsense, because you should eat carbs before bed?

Oh, and there is more confusion to add. What (fad) diet should you use? Should you try the SlimFast diet, because they claim to be "America's #1 favorite weight loss plan"[1] and the easiest and fastest way to lose weight? For the record, fast weight loss is not healthy. I'll touch on that more in later chapters. For now, let's go back to what causes confusion. You may have read that Paleo is better for you, because you eat like cavemen, and that gluten is bad; therefore, do not eat foods that contain it. Which foods are those anyway? Or should you do Weight Watchers, Nutrisystem, or Jenny Craig?

All you want to do is lose weight, and then you want to keep it off—not for a few months, not for a few years—for good. You do not want confusion about how you do it. You just want a process you can follow that helps you lose weight and keep it off for good. Some will say that programs such as Weight Watchers, Nutrisystem, and Jenny Craig offer you that. They most certainly can be used as a guide, as a way to implement healthier habits in your life, and to help you manage your portion sizes. I will not rebut that. I am here, as a living witness, to share with you that you do not need such programs to reach your weight-loss goal or even to maintain your weight after losing it. You can do like me: live diet-free.

---

[1] "SlimFast™ | How It Works." *SlimFast.* SlimFast. Web. 15 May 2016. http://slimfast.ca/how-it-works.

Being successful at weight loss is more than following a plan. It takes being mindful of what you do and why you do it. It also takes embracing the journey, taking in all that it has to offer: learning life lessons, building mental and physical strength, learning to love yourself, being accepting of challenges, and gaining confidence. Not only that, it takes living a process you can sustain for a lifetime. You need what I've realized is required for success with not only losing weight but keeping it off for good.

Several years ago, I gained a significant amount of weight—fifty pounds, to be exact. I lost that weight and kept it off for six years (yay me!), but then I gained upwards of one hundred pounds. (It might have actually been more, but I was avoiding the scale.) Thankfully, I eventually lost that too.

During my weight-loss journey, people often asked, "How did you do it?" I knew—just like you—that losing weight consisted of regular exercise and a nutrient-rich, healthy diet. That is how I kept the weight off for those six years. What I did *not* know resulted in me gaining the weight back, plus some. So, that is what I will share in this book. It relates to not only what you eat but also understanding why we struggle to stay on the weight-loss journey as well as the importance of planning and preparation for success in losing weight and keeping it off.

I wrote this book because so many people in my daily path were asking me the question, "How did you do it?" as they witnessed my physical change. This book is for the coworker who stopped me in the elevator and asked, "Did you do it by only eating salad, because I don't like salad?" (And no, I did not only eat salad. As my nephew put it, I ate *food* food.) It is for the single mother who wanted to know if I take a cheat day. This book is for the woman who has been struggling to lose weight and asked me for help. It's for the cousin who waited for me to leave a party and told me privately that she needed to stop gaining weight but was at her wit's end. *Diet-Free Me* is for all the people who said, "I see you are still on a diet," (when I never was) and to those who wondered aloud when I was going to stop eating "that way" (healthy), since I had already lost weight. Most importantly, *Diet-Free Me* is for anyone who has yet to discover what I realized. To even begin living your weight-loss journey requires a change in how you think. The process begins in your mind. It begins when you dig deep down into understanding why you behave the way you do when it comes to eating. From there, it is understanding how vital planning and preparation are to your success. Even if you go off track, you can correct it by realizing what is happening and making the necessary adjustments before falling too far.

If you need to lose weight, if you are sick and tired of dieting, if you have had enough of the vicious cycle of gaining and losing and gaining weight again (plus some), if you don't need to lose weight but want to be healthier, if you want to maintain your current weight, or if you want to hear from someone who has successfully reached a goal and wonder, "How'd You Do It?" keep reading to see what is in store for you.

The next pages will guide you through the key to that success. The focus of this book is to share how I handled eating along my journey of losing seventy-five pounds. It is about how I learned to structure my eating such that I am no longer the woman who hates how she looks in the mirror, with no confidence in herself. Primarily, it is about realizing what I need to do in order to never go back to being that woman again.

I want to make this clear: This is not a diet book. There will be no mention of me having used fad diets here. There are no references to diet pills, plastic body wraps, or plastic body suits, and there will be no mention of me sitting in a sauna for hours at a time. This book answers those questions and cries for help that I encountered along my journey. I share that information in a relatable, easy-to-follow, and—I hope—fun way.

This book, then, is me answering the question, "How did I do it?" I want to show you that you are capable of achieving weight-loss success without becoming a nutritionist, fitness instructor, or dietitian. All you have to be is you, the person who wants to see changes in life by becoming healthier, by losing weight in the process, and by having the frame of mind to keep it off for a lifetime.

This is meant to be a guide. Start by reading the first four chapters: "Chapter 1: The First Time Was Bad; the Second Didn't Last; the Third Time Nearly Broke Me," "Chapter 2: When You Have Had Enough, Dig Deep into Your *Why?*" "Chapter 3: Get That C.R.A.P. Out of My House," and "Chapter 4: Don't Be Caught with Your Pants Down —Be Prepared." After reading those chapters, have at it. Read the chapters that are appropriate for you in any order that you please. Reading them in order, however, probably makes the most sense. Here is an overview of the chapters to give you an idea of what is ahead.

How'd You Do It? The Breakdown of Each Chapter

Diet-Free Me is comprised of twelve chapters that share how I successfully lost weight, including the strategies I still use to make sure I never again relapse. It explains what you can do too, modifying it to fit your needs, your likes, your biology, and your life, as everyone's experience differs and one size does not fit all. Since this book is about a healthy lifestyle, you have the freedom to use trial and error to determine what does and does not work for you.

Chapter 1: The First Time Was Bad; the Second Time Nearly Broke Me. I tell the stories of what led me to gain a significant amount of weight, not once but twice. It also shares how I lost that weight both times and how, after the second time, I was left asking myself a very important question: "How will I be certain that this time I make sure this never happens again?"

Chapter 2: When You Have Had Enough, Dig Deep into Your *Why?* I guide you through the process that had the greatest impact on my life. It is the process I used to finally break the cycle of losing weight and gaining it back. You must—I repeat, you must—understand your triggers and behaviors, not only for this book to work for you but, I believe, to be successful at any life change. Without this foundation, you will not be prepared for when life happens.

Chapter 3: Get That C.R.A.P. Out of My House. I take you through the process of cleaning out your life and home of foods that will work against you. The chapter is not about depriving you of food but thinking of certain foods like bad relationships. You have choices: completely break up, make compromises through adjustments, or keep them around, only partaking in moderation.

Chapter 4: Don't Be Caught with Your Pants Down—Be Prepared. I share with you what happens when we are not prepared, whether that be for life changes or planning ahead. I then give you suggestions for how to be prepared, plan ahead, or at least understand why planning and preparation are so important to your success.

Chapter 5: Tools of the Trade—the Go-To Technology. I share two applications. I used one to track the calories I burned through exercise and normal, everyday activity as well as my food intake, specifically the calories and nutritional information. The other provided pertinent nutritional information about the food I had eaten, had planned to eat, or had planned to purchase.

Chapter 6: From Grocery-Shopping Flunky to Master Shopper. This chapter arms you with strategies for making it through the grocery-shopping process with foods that will work in your best interest, even if you hate grocery shopping.

Chapter 7: Don't Be Fooled. Once you have a strategy for grocery shopping, for optimal success you need to understand what you are eating. In this chapter, I make sure that you are not fooled by tricky and untrustworthy marketing.

Chapter 8: Water Does a Body and Mind Good. What we drink is as essential to our weight-loss success as what we eat. If there is anything that we must drink, it is water. I share the benefits of water as well as ideas for getting enough water each day. I also share ideas for those who do not like water.

Chapter 9: Putting it All Together. In this chapter, I combine all of the prior chapters into one, showing you how I work them all together in my life.

Chapter 10: Tips, Tricks, and *Oh No I Won't.* As you succeed along your weight-loss journey, you will hit bumps in the road, distractions, tantalizing temptations, and compromising situations. This chapter readies you to deal with those challenges.

Chapter 11: Move Your Body! To supplement the lifestyle change in your eating habits, I recommend levels of exercise, ideas for setting your workout schedule and frequency, and how to squeeze in a workout when your schedule refuses to allow it.

Chapter 12: And, in Conclusion, Make Sure You Stay on Top. The purpose of this book is to share what I did to lose weight and what I do to maintain it and regroup when life challenges arise. This final chapter concludes with setting the reminder that the goal is more than losing weight—it's about living a lifestyle that will allow you to be healthy and confident for a lifetime.

The Struggle Is Real

Within each of the above chapters, I compiled all that I did to reach my weight-loss success and what I do to live a healthier lifestyle. I consider that information the "How To Do It" information. But I did not stop there.

I know firsthand that the weight-loss struggle is real. We have temptations, procrastination, excuses, and exasperation to contend with as well. That's why—where applicable and based on my own experience, observations, discussions, and questions others have asked me—I included a section called, "Keeping-It-Real Solutions and Helpful Tips for Your Struggles, Challenges, and Excuses."

Your Journey to a Diet-Free Me Starts Now

Let's now begin your journey toward losing weight and ensuring you are prepared to keep it off for good, allowing you to be more confident, feel good about yourself, love the skin that you are in, and walk boldly and proudly.

The hope for this book is to put you in the position where others ask, "How did you do it, and how have you done it for so long?" with no pills, body wraps, saunas, plastic suits, or fad diets.

Let's see exactly how I did this so you can do it too. Are you ready?

Acknowledge that
you're broken;
then begin living a life
that will mend the pieces.

CHAPTER 1

The First Time Was Bad; The Second Didn't Last; And The Third Time Nearly Broke Me

I am sure you are aware of how the story goes. You go on a diet. Then life happens. When it does, it seems to always happen before you reach your weight-loss goal. Ultimately, you stop the diet and stop losing weight. Or maybe you were one of the successful people, able to sustain the constraints of the diet, allowing you to lose all that you wanted to lose. You then stop the diet. Heck, you reached your goal, so why do you need to continue eating that way? A few weeks, months, or even a year—or two or three years—later, you find yourself starting the cycle over again. Why? Because you were not properly prepared for what you need to do to keep the weight off. I am living proof of this very notion.

The First Time Life Happened

In high school, I hated computer programming. For some reason, unlike with math, I simply could not grasp it. Back then, we did not have "friendly" programming languages (Visual Basic), as I like to call them. It was done in programming languages, such as Fortran, Pascal, and COBOL. All of it was completely foreign to me. Truth be told, they made me feel like I was not all that bright. Eight years after graduating college with a psychology degree, a work project in a field unrelated to my degree gave me a new appreciation for computer programming.

I appreciated it so much that I wanted to learn more and use computer programming to help develop more efficient processes for work. To accomplish this, I enrolled in a two-year computer programming curriculum at The Chubb Institute. That was around 1999, too long ago to recall the precise time.

A couple of nights per week, after work, I would commute an hour and twenty minutes from Manhattan to the school in my home state of New Jersey. Class let out around 10:00 p.m., when I would grab something quick to eat, and then head home to work on an assignment or study. Usually too exhausted after a full day at work, followed by three hours of coursework, unable to think about anything else, I went for anything conveniently located near the school. My meals of choice, therefore, were pizza, TGI Fridays Sesame Jack Chicken Strips (which were fried to a golden brown, coated with an Asian panko breading, covered in their signature Jack Daniel's glaze, and then topped with toasted sesame seeds), or two pieces of fried chicken from Kentucky Fried Chicken (KFC). In addition to those wonderful eating habits, I recall several times during that two-year span when I stayed up until 4:00 in the morning to complete a major project, slept for about an hour, and then got ready for another work day.

There is something else important to note. If you have an office job, you know all about this. At the time I was taking these courses, I was in my early thirties. At work, I sat at a desk all day, behind a computer. I was not exercising, unless you count the .6-mile walk from the train station to my office building. I did, but the nurse at work disagreed. At least, it was not enough to make much of a difference, since I was doing nothing else. Besides, who had time for exercise with work, class, and the associated coursework?

That is how I got my first lesson in the evils of aging, a slowing metabolism, and living a sedentary lifestyle while also eating poorly and living on very little sleep. What I ate most of my life, prior to that time, used to have no effect on me whatsoever, but now it was sticking to me, refusing to leave, much like an unwanted guest.

The Results When Life Happened the First Time

As a result, by the time I had completed my coursework in computer programming, I found myself in unfamiliar territory. For the first time in my life, I was overweight. And we are not talking about ten or fifteen pounds either. By the time the program concluded, I had gained fifty pounds! The increase in clothing size over the course of that time was a dead giveaway, but I was still shocked that I had managed to reach that point.

I did not like that I had gained weight. I had never in my life been that size. Prior to that, the most I had ever gained was the "Freshman 15" in college, which I quickly lost during my sophomore year as a walk-on with the Rutgers women's basketball team. Though the weight bothered me, it was not until the day a security guard at work asked me if I were pregnant that I truly had my feelings hurt and was brought to tears once I was alone to shed them.

The Response to When Life Happened the First Time

Not too long after that incident, I sought options to lose weight in a healthy way. I had witnessed work colleagues, family members, and famous people losing weight and relapsing. I wanted to be sure that I did not follow the same path. In my search, I found a book by Bill Phillips, called *Body for Life: 12 Weeks to Mental and Physical Strength*. It was from this book that I learned the difference between dieting and living a healthy lifestyle.

In a nutshell, a diet is what you do only for a period of time. It is has no permanent shelf life. Its very essence is temporary. Why is that? Diets say that for the next X number of days or weeks—it is never too long, twelve weeks max—I will restrict myself to the rules of this diet with the goal of losing however many pounds I am promised to lose. When that time frame is over, if you managed to make it to the end of the program, you are done with the diet and back to life as usual—no more restrictions, no more deprivation. This behavior happens because such restrictions are difficult to sustain for a long period of time. In the process of these diets appealing to our "make it quick and easy," microwave society sensibilities, not only are we deprived of foods, but we are also likely restricted from consuming fats, carbs, and the vitamins and minerals our bodies needs. None of that is healthy. Also, before you know it, in no time at all, you are back to where you started, before the diet. You feel frustrated and eventually give up and go back to habits of eating foods that do not offer nutritious value, like potato chips, fried chicken, and cake.

On the flip side, a healthy lifestyle is something we live every day for the rest of our lives, not for thirty days or twelve weeks, and it isn't about food deprivation. *The Merriam-Webster Dictionary* "simple definition of *lifestyle*" is "a particular way of living: the way a person lives or a group of people live."[2] For *healthy*, the same dictionary has "having good health: not sick or injured; showing good health; or good for your health,"[3] where *health* means, "the condition of being well or free from disease; the overall condition

---

[2] "Lifestyle." *Merriam-Webster*. Merriam-Webster, Incorporated. Web. 27 March 2016. http://www.merriam-webster.com/dictionary/lifestyle.

[3] "Healthy." *Merriam-Webster*. Merriam-Webster, Incorporated. Web. 27 March 2016. http://www.merriam-webster.com/dictionary/healthy.

of someone's body or mind; or the condition or state of something."[4] Thus, living a healthy lifestyle can be said to mean the way in which we live our lives that is good for our health, which includes our minds and our bodies. The goal—our goal—is to stop the battle between gaining and losing weight. Once you lose the weight, the goal is to maintain a lifestyle that will allow you to keep it off. That was the type of life I wanted to live. Thus, I proclaimed that I was not on a diet but rather that I was going to live a healthy lifestyle.

Starting in November 2001, with the combination of eating five or six relatively healthy meals per day, allowing myself a cheat meal on Sundays (I have abandoned that way of thinking), and doing strength training and cardio workouts, mostly in the form of running, five or six times per week, within five months I lost those fifty pounds. That was an average weight loss of ten pounds per month, which, based on the Mayo Clinic's recommended one to two pounds per week, was a healthy and safe weight-loss pace. I did exactly what I said I would do too: I lived a healthy lifestyle. That routine did not end in May of 2002, after losing those fifty pounds. I lived my life following that same prescription for years—until a life change happened.

The Second Time Life Happened

Desiring an addition to my professional credentials once again, I entered graduate school in the fall of 2007. I was still working full-time with the same employer in New York City (NYC). I was still commuting from New Jersey into NYC each day. But, this time, my commute included an additional twenty minutes, making it an hour and forty minutes each way. In addition, I was ten years older than I had been the first time.

With the demands of my job and coursework, I was back to getting little sleep. Eventually, I returned to other old bad habits too. I ate poorly (more on that in "Chapter 3: Get That C.R.A.P. Out of My House") more

---

[4] "Health." *Merriam-Webster.* Merriam-Webster, Incorporated. Web. 27 March 2016. http://www.merriam-webster.com/dictionary/health.

often than I ate healthy. My exercise routine had ceased, making me completely sedentary again. Now ten years older, it seemed as if my metabolism had not only slowed down but that it had completely stopped functioning.

The Results When Life Happened—Again

With a full-time job and being in a program that did not offer summer classes, it took me four years to finish my graduate studies. By the end of the four years, I had a Master's degree, along with weighing an additional hundred pounds. I may have gained more during that time, but I avoided the scale as much as possible; thus, the most I was aware of was one hundred pounds.

I was not only the heaviest I had ever been, but I was also the saddest that I had ever been in my life. Smiling photos did not show it, but I was mentally broken. I hated who I had become. I hated the sight of me when I looked in the mirror. I cried in dressing rooms. I hid away from friends I had not seen but with whom I used to run half-marathons and ski, on occasion.

I knew better. How, then, could I have let that happen—again? And how could I have gained so much more weight?! I asked myself that very question every time I had to buy a bigger size. Somehow, during that period of time, I did not make the appropriate adjustments, even with the knowledge that I had about living a healthy lifestyle.

A Start to Responding When Life Happened—Again

Tired of wallowing in my sorrows, in late 2012, I began the journey of losing weight again. I got back into running. I became mindful of what I ate. By early 2013, I had lost fifty pounds. That left me with another fifty pounds to reach my pre-graduate school weight and return to living a healthy lifestyle.

Life Happening Starts Again?!

Life happened—again. At the same time that I was (once again) not promoted, messing with my head and making me believe I was not good enough, I was also doing somewhat of a road show. My goal was to get to the stage and become the World Champion of Public Speaking within Toastmasters International. For several weeks, I rehearsed, presented, and gave my contest speech. At the third level of the contest, the Division Contest, which would put me two steps closer to the World Championship stage, I gave the same speech I had given up to that point. Much to the shock of many in attendance, and myself, I did not win the contest that night. In fact, I somehow managed to not even place in the top three.

All that preparation had led to a loss. For months, I listened to people telling me how confused they were. Imagine how I felt. Between the overwhelming self-doubt from not getting promoted and the many nights of preparing for what I had hoped would make me a speaking celebrity, even if it was only within the Toastmasters community, I was hurt. When I was hurt, I needed comfort. That comfort came from food.

More Undesirable Results without Motivation to Try Again

That fifty-pound loss fizzled away. In short order, I had gained back twenty-five of those fifty pounds. During the remainder of that year (2013) and the beginning of 2014, I tried getting back on track, but the desire to do what needed to be done—eat healthy and work out regularly—simply was not in me. I knew how much discipline and hard work it took to lose weight after the programming courses. The mere thought of that seemed to make me want to eat more just to feel good, even if only for a moment.

In July of 2014, I went on my wedding anniversary trip to San Francisco. During that trip, we did a lot of walking up those massive hills, not as a form of predetermined exercise but because we had opted for public transportation over renting a car as a way to save money. Using public transportation sometimes meant walking. In addition, we also did our fair share of getting our grub on with not-so-healthy choices. Talk about letting myself go.

Enough, You Need to Change

After returning home from the vacation, I was looking at photos from our trip. One photo struck me hard. I cannot tell you why this particular photo, and none prior, hit me the way that it did. But that photo of me in a light-orange warm-up jacket, on a boat leaving the Fisherman's Wharf and heading to Alcatraz, made me say to myself, "Enough. You need to change."

That was the day my life changed. Soon after, I found a personal trainer via a Google search (Oh, how I love Google.) But, before I did a search for a personal trainer, I did something I had not done before starting the computer programming classes or graduate school. I took the time to ask myself how I managed to get to the point that I gained fifty—then one hundred—pounds. Then I asked myself the most important question of all: *How will I be certain that this time I make sure it never happens again?*

It is from the basis of that question that I wrote this book. If you have been struggling to eat your way to a lifetime of weight loss, the next chapters will act as your guide to show you where to place your focus.

HOW TO DO IT

Read the next three chapters. Do not skip them. These chapters helped me get on track.

Decide how you will proceed with the book. After the first three chapters, the order in which you read the book does not matter—only the content does. You can continue reading in order, or you can jump back to the "Table of Contents" to determine your next step. Along my journey, I used all of

18

these methods to help me lose those seventy-five pounds. No matter how much weight you need to lose, these chapters will help make a difference.

Keep the book handy at all times. Consider it your reminder and your accountability partner.

Tell others about your goal. Reach out to like-minded people or to people who want to accomplish the same goals as you. Reach out to people who really are ready to change their lives—for life. These are the people who will act as your advisor, your coach, or push you when you need it.

Stay connected with your accountability partner on a consistent and regular basis. A key to success with any goal is having someone who will hold you accountable. To make that partnership more effective, you must be certain that you are consistent with your interaction with that partner. After telling them what you desire to do, decide on the method you will use to communicate, and then set the frequency of that communication. For example, on days I did not work out with my personal trainer, I sent her an email to let her know what workout I had done without her. The email included what I did, when I did it, and for how long. In your case, you can share what you eat each day.

Move on to the next chapter. There I will guide you through the process that had the greatest impact on my life. It is the process I used to be certain that I break the cycle of losing weight and gaining it back.

Know why you do
what you do
to begin changing
what you do.

CHAPTER 2

WHEN YOU HAVE HAD ENOUGH, DIG DEEP INTO YOUR *WHY?*

Aha!

Exercise and eating healthy are keys to losing weight, yes. More important, I realized, is what you do when you have reached your weight-loss goal, when life happens, when the unexpected arises, or when your responsibilities and goals change. We can avoid major setbacks, relapses, and the feeling of being broken when we understand why we do what we do and are prepared for it. This was the pivotal "aha!" moment that spoke to me, because, when I lost the weight that next time, I would be sure to keep it off for a lifetime.

I sat at my computer, looking through photos we had taken on our trip to San Francisco. Amongst the photos of tourist points, such as the Golden Gate Bridge, Muir Woods National Monument, the Fisherman's Wharf, and Alcatraz, were pictures of me. One photo, in particular, stopped my steady flow of reminiscing through our time in San Francisco.

Attention Grabber

What had caught my attention? Looking back at me was a picture of me. In the photo, I was standing in my newly purchased orange warm-up jacket, the one I bought the night before leaving for the trip, because I had outgrown my clothes from the previous trip only a couple of months prior. My face was round, almost looking puffy, and a couple of other things (wink wink) had gotten large too.

Over the three to four years prior to that photo, I had many others where I look about the same. There may have been some variations of me being bigger or slightly smaller, but there was nothing significantly different about me in that picture compared with the others. The only clear difference was my reaction to seeing the photo.

The furrowing of my brows was the same. The disgust with myself for getting to that point was the same. What was different was that, in that moment, as the eyes in that photo looked back at me with a slight smile, I had finally gotten to the point of having enough of me. I wish I could tell you what it was about that day, about that photo, that brought the change in me. I honestly cannot tell you. All I can tell you is, like the words of Fannie Lou Hamer, I had gotten sick and tired of me being sick and tired of me.

That Moment When You've Had Enough of You

But something more happened in that moment. I did not simply say to myself that I needed to change what I was currently doing. At that time, I was doing nothing of what I knew needed to be done to change my situation. I had traveled the weight-gain to weight-loss road before. I knew I needed to exercise and stop eating like I had no sense. I determined that I needed to not only lose weight but make certain that this time I never ever, ever gain it back again.

Know What's Really Going on with You

That is the point you will have to reach as well. It is not enough to decide you will lose weight and start exercising and changing what you eat. You must be prepared for what losing weight and keeping it off entails. You have to understand the behaviors you possess that got you where you are now. You have to understand what triggers those behaviors. You also need to be sure you understand when your behaviors and triggers hit. Armed with this knowledge about yourself, you will be well on your way to making your weight-loss outcome last a lifetime.

HOW TO DO IT

Do not skip this part! If you want to benefit from this book and lose weight for a lifetime, which I believe that you do since you are reading it, please do not cheat yourself by skipping this part. I know you are anxious for the tools to help you lose weight, but this section is the most important part. It is what you will have to come back to time and time again throughout your life. This section will be the difference between repeating the weight-loss/weight-gain cycle and living a life of never gaining weight again. You'll need it again and again, because, for as long as you live, you will be faced with life challenges and changes of circumstance. Understanding and knowing the steps that follow will help prepare you to react accordingly in those moments. Even if you fall off track, because this chapter will arm you with a better understanding of yourself, you will know how to adjust and what to adjust, and you will be able to adjust a whole lot faster than in the past, thus putting you back on track before you lose control. Are we good? Awesome! Now, on to the next step.

Identify and write down every moment, event, or situation in your life that is related to your weight. What you are looking for here are patterns. Think about or look back to Chapter 1, where I shared three stories related to my weight gain after furthering my education and career credentials. Those were pivotal moments in my life where I gained significant weight. You do not have to have gained as much weight as I did for this assessment. The goal is to identify what situations and circumstances and when you have a tendency to fall off track and stay off, or gain weight. At pamelaburke.com/dietfreeme-resources, I have listed some possible life events to spark your thinking.

Write down your emotional state for each of those life events. How did you feel? Were you sad, anxious, worried, or mentally and physically fatigued? Whatever you felt during that time, write it down. I, for instance, had put a great deal of pressure on myself to get good grades while in both the computer programming courses and in graduate school. Accomplishing that while working full-time made me feel anxious and stressed. In addition, because I had gotten into the habit of staying up late to complete projects and coursework, I also was extremely tired most of the day.

Identify and write down your reactions to your emotional state. You may need to think hard about this, because you may not have realized that you had taken on certain behaviors as a result of your emotional state. At the time that I was taking those courses, I did not realize it, hence the reason I became so far gone. To deal with the anxiety, stress, and sleep deprivation, I sought out comfort to make me feel better. I found that comfort in chocolate candy, fried chicken after class, and other fattening foods lacking nutritional value.

Continuously review your relationship with food. As you read further in the book, you will see more about how food relates to certain situations in my life. When your memory is sparked, go back to the lists you wrote above and add to them or modify them accordingly. You will be amazed how much you will learn that your mental state affects your reaction to food and your waistline.

Take ten to fifteen minutes to get started with the above steps, and then continue on to the next chapter. There I will guide you through your breakup or change in relationship with the foods that do you no good.

Garbage in,
garbage out,
so keep the garbage
out of your mouth.

CHAPTER 3

GET THAT C.R.A.P.
OUT OF MY HOUSE

Do you have favorite foods—those foods that you could eat and eat and eat, never getting tired of them? You only stop eating them because you become overly full. I have a few favorites. Most of them consist of some form of simple carbohydrate, those that are loaded with sugar. That includes sweets, chocolate candy, macaroni and cheese, and, my all-time favorite, bread—especially white flour breads.

I will never forget when Dunkin' Donuts introduced the twists line. They started with about three varieties, but the one that has hung around to this day made me weak: the cheddar cheese bagel twist. I easily went to Dunkin' three times a day to have my cheddar cheese bagel twist. It was a bread addiction like no other.

Mom's Macaroni and Cheese

Thankfully, Mom's macaroni and cheese was not readily available to me. Think of an ice cream scoop. I estimate that I would have three scoops of her

27

mac and cheese, often going back for seconds—that was usually only about two scoops. (I chuckle now.)

Fried Chicken and Waffles

I already had a liking of waffles. It's like a bread, after all. But fried chicken and waffles? It was not until a trip to Atlanta for a Women's NCAA Final Four Basketball tournament that I was introduced to chicken and waffles. While there, we decided to give Gladys Knight's Chicken and Waffles a visit. I was skeptical at first about this particular food combination. I had never heard of such a thing before that day. In fact, I thought the combination was quite odd. That was until I tried it. Fried chicken and waffles—I was in heaven.

Thank goodness, three things were going for me back then. For one, living in the Northeast, unless I made them (which I was not going to do, because I do not cook), at that time, finding a restaurant that served fried chicken and waffles was going to be a challenge. Second, being that my mom and aunts are from the South, they offered possible alternatives to finding a restaurant, but, since I had never heard of the chicken-and-waffles combination prior to that trip, I did not suspect any of them were going to start making chicken and waffles simply because I requested them. I was in the clear. Third, at that time in my life, it did not matter much that chicken and waffles were not readily available. I was still well into my healthy lifestyle from my first weight-loss journey. I was so disciplined with my eating that I had no plans of making that type of meal a habit.

That all changed during my graduate school years. I recall running into our pastor and his family at a barbecue place in Newark, NJ, called Dinosaur. I had settled for barbecue, but what I really wanted that day was fried chicken with a really good Belgian waffle. I mentioned this craving to the pastor and his family. The youngest daughter referred me to a diner in East Newark, NJ, called Tops Diner, which is one of the best diners in New Jersey, for the record. (When in New Jersey, be sure to go to Tops. Flip to the healthy options page, where they have some really great choices. The service is also top-notch.)

The following Sunday, I was fiending (Urban Dictionary: To deeply and uncontrollably miss something or someone[5]) for chicken and waffles again. Recall that, during the graduate school years, I had ditched my healthy eating and regular exercise routine. You know what I did, right? That Sunday, after church, I decided to visit Tops to give their chicken and waffles a try. Oh. WOW! The experience was heavenly. The chicken was moist, without being greasy. The waffles were light and airy with a slight taste of sweetness.

It was all over after that initial visit to Tops. The only thing that kept the trips there from being more frequent was that the diner was not near home. That made Sundays after church the only time we would go to the restaurant. Another reason was because there were only so many Sundays in a row that I wanted to wait twenty-five or more minutes to eat. Thank goodness for that too, because a half-chicken (you read that correctly) and a waffle a week would have caused collateral damage. For the record, even though I was off the healthy eating routine, I would have never eaten half a chicken. I always started with the juiciest pieces, the dark meat—the thigh and leg. I was usually too full to eat more than that. It also helped that wings are my least favorite part of the chicken.

Let Go of the C.R.A.P.

Bread, macaroni and cheese, sugary treats, and fried chicken were my favorite foods. To change my lifestyle, though, something had to give. Some of these foods and I had to break up. For other foods, we needed to adjust our relationship and not see each other quite as often. That is why, in this chapter, we work on getting C.R.A.P.—carbonated drinks, refined sugars, artificial foods, and processed foods—out of our lives.

[5] "Fiending." *Urban Dictionary*. Urban Dictionary. Web. 23 May 2016.

PAMELA BURKE

HOW TO DO IT

Divide your favorite foods into three categories: dump, compromise, and keep. What you put in each category is your choice. Your goal is to be honest with yourself about your favorite or go-to foods in your life that you should dump for good, that you can keep around but make a compromise to modify how and when you will partake of them, and that you know are good enough for you that you can keep them around for good. When I did this exercise for myself, I dumped soda and other sugary drinks, such as fruit punch, for good. I have not had soda in ten years. I don't miss it either.

Some foods were not easy to dump for good. Since I knew that, I modified how I have them. I would be fooling myself to think I could stop eating bread altogether. Hence, I never tried. Instead, I modified my intake of it. When I am at my best (I say this because I am not perfect with it), I choose breads that are 100-percent whole grain, and I eat them sparingly. If I go out to a restaurant (again, when I am at my best), I go there telling myself to ask the waiter not to serve bread. I have to do this, because I know bread is my weakness. Sometimes, especially if I am dining with others, I will have the bread, but sharing it at least keeps me from eating as much.

Clear your counters, cabinets, and refrigerator of the foods that add fat and lack nutritional value. In addition to deciding which of your favorite or go-to foods you should eliminate from your life, giving your home a clean sweep will help with your life change and weight-loss success. The types of foods you should remove from your home include processed foods, such as potato chips, as well as cookies, simple carbohydrates, and white breads and pastas. Simple carbohydrates, if you do not know, are sugars. Some foods that are considered simple carbohydrates will be familiar to you, including table sugar, brown sugar, corn syrup, fruit drinks, soda, and candy.

I mentioned in the first step how I handle bread, which you should know by now is one of my favorite foods. Get this: the only bread I keep in my house, if I buy bread at all, is Sprouted 100% Whole Grain Ezekiel bread. It

30

does not contain added sugars like other breads. Ezekiel bread is made from sprouted grains, consisting of six grains and legumes: wheat, barley, soybeans, lentils, millet, and spelt. Since I know bread is my weakness, it is best for me not to have it around.

Go to pamelaburke.com/dietfreeme-resources for a listing of the types of foods to start removing from your home in exchange for healthier options. You will want to do this because, by not keeping these items in your house, you will avoid the risk of temptation and splurging. Don't faint and do not believe that will leave you with nothing to eat. You will have plenty to eat. Your options will be different yet flavorful.

Replace what you got rid of above with nutrient-rich foods and complex carbohydrates. It may seem like, by the time you clear your home of the "not good for you/stick to your bones" types of foods, you will be left with barely more than spices. That is not the case. Here you will get used to stocking your home with better alternatives. Check the pamelaburke.com/dietfreeme-resources website for the types of foods that should be in your shopping cart. In "Chapter 6: From Grocery-Shopping Flunky to Master Shopper," you will learn strategies for the grocery-shopping experience.

Move forward to planning and preparation. In the next chapter, we will focus on planning and preparation. You have already started this process by replacing foods with better options.

Keeping-It-Real Solutions and Helpful Tips for Your Struggles, Challenges, and Excuses

I can't let go of the flavor/sugar that makes it taste so good. When I was fifteen years old, my mother took me to work with her one day. I found it odd that she would take me out of school, but I did not question her. Later that afternoon, I learned that my mother had tricked me into thinking I was going to her job to help with some of her work. The real reason for the trip to work, which was in a hospital, was to get blood drawn. She knew how deathly afraid of needles I was. I am slightly better now; I get through the process by closing my eyes and turning my head away. On that afternoon, though, it took my mother, two nurses, and the doctor to hold me down. My mother tells the story like this: "If that wall was not behind her, that fool would have gone running out of the office." I was not pleased with my mother for tricking me. In the end, however, that trip saved my life. At fifteen years old, even though I was rail thin, I had high blood pressure. I was much too young to be suffering from high blood pressure. I understood how it happened. I put salt on practically everything without testing if the food even needed salt. I put salt on pizza, including pepperoni, essentially turning it into a salt lick. After my diagnosis, I kept the salt shaker on the table. The more I did not add salt, the more I could taste the food. In fact, to this day, I am salt sensitive. What seems perfectly fine to someone who likes adding salt to their food tastes too salty to me.

What I am trying to tell you is that, with both salt and sugar, as you cut back, you will find that you do not want or need them. You will also find that most foods taste fine without them. I say most foods, because I will admit that seasoning does add flavor. I encourage you to use alternative options to produce that flavor. In "Chapter 9: Putting it All Together," I go into more detail about alternatives in the "How to Do It" section of that chapter.

I am not always sure what the better options are. I sometimes do not know the better options either. A great deal of what I share with you in *Diet-Free Me* is what I learned from years of looking for answers. It may be cliché, but knowledge is power. With information constantly being updated on the Internet, there is plenty of information available to us for learning about and finding better options. I will warn you, however, that not all information is good information. As I stated in "Introduction: You Most Certainly Are Not Alone," people have opinions about everything. I cut through that noise by consulting with websites, such as www.mayoclinic.org and www.webmd.com.

If you need an alternative for a product, check out "Chapter 5: Tools of the Trade—the Go-To Technology." In that chapter, I share an application I use to help me look for alternative options for products. When it comes to recipes, if I find myself raising an eyebrow at an ingredient, I will search for a healthier alternative. For example, did you know that there are natural alternatives for butter? When I wanted a substitution for butter, I did it through a Google search and by checking Pinterest. In doing so, I found alternatives like applesauce and extra virgin coconut oil. I also learned that you need to know whether those alternatives are best for baking or switching out for a meal you are cooking.

With regard to sugar, I do not add it to food. I used to order my coffee light and sweet. To make the change, I slowly modified how I order it. First, I started by reducing the size from a medium to a small. After about a week or two, I would order a small coffee with skim milk and one sugar. I then progressed to no sugar. I have been ordering my coffee without sugar for sixteen years now. I recently ordered a cup of coffee, without sugar. I sipped it, as it was hot, and nearly spit it out all over my living room table, not because it was hot but because it was sweet. I wanted my morning coffee, but there was no way in the world I could drink it. My palate had changed so much over the years that I could not stand having something so sweet. Frustrated, I went back to Dunkin' Donuts and asked for a new coffee. The young man who had made it confirmed that he had added the sugar, even though I had not ordered it, because he had never heard of anyone ordering coffee without sugar. (Eye-roll.)

Small Changes Make a Huge Difference

Trust me, by taking one step at a time and making slow modifications, you will learn that you do not need the added salt or sugar either. Keep this at the forefront of your mind: It is not that you cannot eat certain foods; you are now making the healthier choice not to eat certain foods. If you want a better handle on what you eat, you can start by making sure you are always prepared. We discuss planning and preparation in the next chapter.

Always keep at the forefront
of your mind that by being
prepared you are ultimately
prepared.

CHAPTER 4

DON'T BE CAUGHT WITH YOUR PANTS DOWN—BE PREPARED

At this point, you know that the goal of this book is to save you from reliving the cycle of losing weight to only gain it back again. You also know that you need more than regular exercise and diet to help in that success. In your understanding of this, you now have an awareness of your relationship with food as a result of life events and your various emotional states throughout life. Equipped with the information you have gathered about yourself, you are now better prepared to handle such circumstances and feelings. Finally, in the last chapter, you began changing your relationship with food. There are some foods that you have eliminated from your life and others that you have modified when and how you eat them. Now that you have done that, in this chapter, I will guide you through how to plan and be prepared for everyday living, no matter the situation.

Bad Habit Formation and No Plan of Action

As you know from the first two chapters, when I was in graduate school, I was also working full-time. The school was a two-minute walk from my office building. That was a great commute—the commute home, not so much. Including the walk to New York Penn Station, the train ride, and the drive home, my commute was one and a half hours.

During the four years it took me to complete my graduate program, I picked up several really bad eating habits. In the earlier years, before class, I would have a relatively healthy meal. Over time, what I ate before, during, and after class attributed to my tremendous weight gain. Let me also add that all of this was happening while the only exercise I was getting was the twelve- to fifteen-minute walk to and from New York Penn Station. The duration of that walk increased to twenty minutes as I gained weight.

At least two nights a week, I was getting home at 11:00 p.m. or later. On the nights I was not in class, I stayed up late completing an assignment or studying for an exam. As for the poor eating habits, what did that look like?

On the walk to class, I would stop in the nearby bodega and purchase any variety of items, such as Now & Later candies, lollipops, peanuts (I considered those my healthy item), a Kit Kat, or all of the above. In between classes, I sought out the vending machines. There were not many healthy choices in there anyway. Sometimes I got chips or pretzels (my attempt at healthy, considering the options); sometimes I chose Skittles, Twizzlers, a Hershey bar, or a Kit Kat. I like sweet candy, and I love chocolate.

After class, because I am all about routine (or a creature of habit), I would stop at Popeye's Chicken. The order was always the same: a crispy two-piece, dark-meat (leg and thigh) meal with a biscuit and fries. Remember, that was at least two times a week. If I did not have time to stop at Popeye's, I would grab two slices of pizza at the train station.

This is What Happens When You Aren't Prepared

Combining horrible food choices, lack of physical exercise, and lack of sleep (usually four hours or less), by the time I completed graduate school, I went from a size eight to a size twenty-four. As mentioned previously, at my known largest, I had gained one hundred pounds. All of that could have been avoided if I had done one thing: prepare.

Always Be Ready: Practice Planning and Preparation for Any Situation

As mentioned in "Chapter 2: When You Have Had Enough, Dig Deep into Your *Why?*" situations come up in life. Some of those situations and circumstances sneak up on us: the unexpected loss of a loved one, the loss of a job, a change in job responsibilities and/or work hours, or maybe a shift in home life, such as taking care of elderly parents who have regressed to the point they seem like your children. We all have different stories. Such situations may require an adjustment period. What is important, regardless of the circumstance, is to not lose sight of your greater priority: you. Without you at your healthy best, you are no good for anyone else. Put into practice the planning and preparation of what you will eat. That is the best way to protect yourself from getting into a position similar to where I found myself after graduate school.

HOW TO DO IT

Prepare your own meals. Yes, I was crazy busy and extremely tired during the time I was in school, but, had I taken the time to prepare my own meals, I would not have fallen into the bad habits I mentioned.

By preparing and bringing your own meals with you, you also save yourself from wandering eyes and temptations. That is, your eyes wander over to that food option you know you probably should not have; you get tempted; then, the next thing you know, you're sitting down, eating it, later deciding that you fell off and might as well keep going off the tracks.

OK, I know that is the worst-case scenario, but I want you thinking about that as a possibility. That is part of your training for changing your habits. As I lost weight and developed better habits, I was less likely to act upon my wandering eyes. I usually walked away with a smile when I noticed what I had done. As you keep at it, choosing healthy habits will become second nature. If you believe that you struggle to find a way or time to prepare, plan, and cook meals, this is the chapter for you. Following are the best ways that I have found to help you be most successful at preparing your own meals:

1. **Plan your meals for the week.** Now that we have you moving in the direction of preparing your own meals, you must now add a pillar to your preparing-your-own-meal success. You do this by planning your meals for the whole week. After you finish planning, move on to the next step, because planning alone is not enough to help you be successful with preparing your own meals.

2. **Dedicate a day for meal preparation.** Not only does preparing your own meals help keep you honest and avoid temptation, but creating a routine for when you cook your meals will bring you much more success than if you do not schedule meal preparation.

   Everyone has their own schedule; therefore, you will have to determine what day and time works best for you. The day that works best for me is Sunday, in the early evening.

3. **Freeze it now for another day.** In our house, there are only two of us. Since I can be so spastic when it comes to the idea of deciding what to eat, I must rely on recipes I find in books or on the Internet. More often than not, those meals are not meant for only two people. One way around that is cutting the ingredients in half. Another option is combining the ingredients as described in the recipe and then freezing the excess.

   I made a ground-turkey meatball recipe once, and it was way too much. Rather than cooking it all, I put some of the mixture in the freezer. A few weeks later, when I was preparing dinner on a Sunday evening, that turkey meatball mixture became one of the meals. The cool thing about it was that, since the ingredients had already been mixed together, I saved a lot of time, which made it easier to prepare two meals to split between lunch and dinner throughout the week.

Keep healthy portable snacks with you at all times. When you go into a convenience store, they conveniently have rows with chips, pastries, and candies. Behind the glass of your local coffee shop are donuts, Danishes, cookies, and croissants. Even at stores like Best Buy and Office Depot, you walk through a maze of gum and candy as you check out. The convenience is good; the choices are dangerous. This is why it is important that you carry your snacks—healthy snacks—with you. In doing so, you will save yourself from unwanted calories that do not benefit you in any way. Refer to pamelaburke.com/dietfreeme-resources for ideas.

Bring food with you when traveling. I mentioned above that you should have healthy portable snacks with you at all times. This includes short trips, personal trips, work-related trips, and vacations. Whether you are taking a road trip or flying, be sure to bring along healthy snacks and meals. Not only will this save you from temptation, it will also save you money, and it will save the hard work you put into decreasing your clothing size.

Place your food in travel containers. Plastic bags work well. For instance, for each day that you will be away, put a scoop of protein powder, almonds, or walnuts into a separate baggie. By planning this way, you have options readily at your disposal, and you control your portion sizes. I will talk more about portion sizes in "Chapter 9: Putting it All Together." Refer to the pamelaburke.com/dietfreeme-resources website for additional ideas.

Keeping-It-Real Solutions and Helpful Tips for Your Struggles, Challenges, and Excuses

Don't have time or you're too tired to prep meals. Hey, I get it. In fact, I hate cooking. However, I have to tell myself that, even for me, it is not an excuse. That means I have to consider alternatives. Here are some "I don't have time to prep meals" solutions:

1. **Have someone prepare the meals for you.** If you are not able to make meals for yourself or can't make the time, invest your money instead. There are companies existing now that will make and deliver meals for you. Since it is so difficult for us to think of recipes on our own, we invest in meals from Home Chef. During the week, we select from the options made available by Home Chef, based on our preferences: low carbohydrates and low-calorie. We then select two to three meals, which are delivered to our doorstep on Fridays. On Sundays, we do our version of acting like the grown ups that we are by preparing the meals based on the ingredients and instructions provided with each meal.

    Another option, if you have the financial means to do so, is to invest in a personal chef.

2. **Find restaurants, eateries, or grocery stores that prepare healthy meals.** Before we invested in Home Chef, I ate out for my meals a lot more often than I do now. Besides the possibility of being expensive, eating out can also be a detriment to your weight-loss and weight-maintenance goals. You have no idea how the food is prepared. Are they using too much salt? What type of oil are they using in the food preparation? Do they add sugar as an ingredient? You really have no idea. In addition, some eateries only offer fattening food options—fried, not baked or grilled. For this reason, if you are going to make eating out a habit, you must be prepared for it. How do you find these places? In "Chapter 5: Tools of the Trade—the Go-To Technology," I will give you tools that I use in helping me be prepared before going out to eat. For now, I will tell you that I purposefully look for places offering healthy options or those which can be modified to be healthier. Another way to find these places is to use Google or Yelp. Using Google, do a search for

"healthy restaurants near me." Google will then return a list of nearby restaurants that they somehow deem healthy. The Healthy Dining Finder website (www.healthydiningfinder.com) has also come up during my searches. When you go to the site, enter your address, zip code, or city. After clicking search, you will get of list of options. For both the Google search results and Healthy Dining Finder results list, I am quick to question their suggestions. I advise that you do the same.

For every restaurant that I am considering, I use the same routine, especially when I find myself questioning what is returned on the search list. Part of that routine is to check the restaurant website, if they have one. Usually, I do not consider a place if they do not have a website. You will understand why in a moment.

When I go to the website, I look for the menu and the nutritional information. Again, more on that in Chapter 5. First, I browse the menu to see what they offer, hoping to find more than a salad as a healthy option; otherwise, I usually move on to a different place. As I mentioned in "Introduction: You Most Certainly Are Not Alone," you do not have to live on salads to lead a healthy lifestyle. Also, I am not really a big fan of them, which is another reason why I would seek out someplace else to eat if that is the only healthy thing they have to offer. Here is my last rant about salads: having one made of iceberg lettuce is a fail, in my book. Of all the leafy greens available, iceberg lettuce ranks the lowest in nutritional value; it is mostly water. Yes, water is a must, as I reference in "Chapter 8: Water Does a Body and Mind Good," but to say that a lettuce consisting of 96-percent water is the only healthy option, to me, is disappointing. Now, if I am out on the road without being prepared and the only thing available to me is McDonald's (or the like), then I am running—not walking—for that salad made with iceberg lettuce. I am sure to keep that salad dressing way off on the side too. I will share a trick that I use for salad dressing in "Chapter 10: Tips, Tricks, and *Oh No I Won't*."

OK, back to my routine. Another thing I look for on the menu is how the food is prepared. I specifically look for baked and grilled options. I watch for the types of proteins that are offered. My main choices are chicken, shrimp, salmon, or some type of white fish, such as cod. I also check what types of vegetables and fruits, if any, are on the menu.

Second to checking the menu is reviewing the nutritional information. Chain restaurants usually do have that information. Be sure to use what I share in Chapter 5 or look at the website for the restaurant you are considering. Those TGI Fridays Sesame Jack Chicken Strips may sound like a healthy option, but those babies contain 1,090 calories and thirty-five grams of fat. When it comes to restaurants that are not a chain, obtaining the nutritional information may be a little more of a challenge. You can call the restaurant and ask if they have one available. If not, that is not the end of the world. This is where you use the opportunity to ask for modifications to the dish. See "Chapter 10: Tips, Tricks, and *Oh No I Won't*," for the types of modifications that you can make to those meals.

You have time to cook, but it takes time to cook. Who you tellin'? After the work day and an almost two-hour commute, the thought of cooking makes me more tired than I already am. I want my meals quick and healthy. Check out other tips here and in the next chapter to see how to deal with the, "If it takes longer than five minutes to make it, that's too long," dilemma.

Do not know what to prepare that is deemed good for the waistline. If you have no problem planning what to eat for the week but have issues with preparing meals that are waistline-slimming friendly, here is what I suggest. Between the Internet and books, there is a wealth of options available to you. Be sure to take advantage of them.

1. **Search for websites that offer suggestions for healthy meals that are quick to make.** I have started searches with "quick healthy meals" using Google. (I LOVE Google!) As I start typing, Google will start guessing

44

what I would like to search. They may suggest "quick healthy dinner meals" or "quick healthy meals for two." Use any one of those searches; then go crazy looking up options from the result set. I personally like the websites that return options for different meal times.

2. **Invest in recipe books.** Kindle on my Apple devices are filled with two genres of books. One is self-help, because I am obsessed with personal growth. The other is related to healthy recipes, such as clean eating, Paleo, green smoothies, and superfoods.

Do not like to cook. I do not like to cook either. That, however, is no reason for not preparing your own meals. I do not enjoy cooking, because I am not a meal-planning visionary. Left to my own devices, I would eat the same thing every day. A lack of variety is not a great way to motivate you to prepare your own meals. To get through this, I follow the same steps as above. I seek out people who love cooking and preparing healthy, clean meals. The most work I have to do is find a recipe that I like and cook it, of course.

Have a family who has no desire to go on this journey with me. We would all hope that, when we do something to change our lives, making us not only physically healthy but also mentally healthy, those we care about and love the most would be encouraging. Sadly, for some of us, that is not the case. Thankfully, this last go around, I had someone in my life who did not need to take the journey but still did it with me. In fact, she lost weight too. I have, however, also had someone in my life who wanted no part of my healthy eating lifestyle. That did not stop me from doing what I needed to do for me. Now, I will admit that, in my case, I was not responsible for anyone else's meals; therefore, it was a little bit easier for me to make meals for myself without having to worry about someone who did not want to partake of what I was eating. For those of you who do not have that support system, I suggest the following:

1. **Make the same type of meals you had been making but with modifications.** In Chapter 10, I will go into this in more detail, but, at a high level, you can change your recipes such that you reduce the fat and sugar.

2. **Stop with the takeout.** By preparing your meals, you stop with the takeout. Reduce or no longer go to fast-food restaurants.

Enough with the Teasing

During this chapter dedicated to planning and preparation, I teased you a bit by mentioning tools that I use to assist with the process. Hold tight, I will get to those tools in a moment. The chapters that follow will no doubt help you gain confidence, but this chapter and those that preceded it will benefit you by helping to prepare you for life's challenges and will help you enjoy weight loss for a lifetime. That is why I advocate for you to reread these earlier chapters. You will want them to really sink in so that you experience optimal results.

Having said that, I am done with the teasing. In the next chapter, I will let you in on my tools of the trade. Those tools are my go-to technology. They served me quite well on my journey to losing seventy-five pounds. Up next is how they can do the same for you.

Take advantage of advanced technology by letting it act as your better health partner.

CHAPTER 5

TOOLS OF THE TRADE— THE GO-TO TECHNOLOGY

So far, these beginning chapters have been about planning and preparation. You started by working on your mental preparation, then moved to your food planning and preparation. In this chapter, we will keep to the planning-and-preparation theme, but now our focus moves to tools you can use to help be on top of your game.

I consider these my tools of the trade—my go-to technology. You will learn how to use this technology to help plan and prepare what and where you eat. These tools also assist you with knowing what not to eat. First, I will take you through what life was like without such technology, then how I used technology to my benefit. Following that is how you too can use my tools of the trade to your benefit.

Not Required but Recommended

When I went on that weight-loss journey in the early 2000s, I did not have these tools at my disposal. I successfully managed to lose the fifty pounds without the need for fancy tools or cool technology. That means what I am about to share with you is not required. Even so, I do recommend it.

As I stated earlier, there was a ten-year time span between when I lost those fifty pounds and when I set out on the journey to losing seventy-five pounds. You are familiar with the grind of everyday life and the aging process. You slow down. Your energy levels are lower. You may lack motivation to do most anything beyond the essentials to get through the day. That was the case for me. I simply did not feel like doing much more than getting up, going to work, coming home to veg out on mindless television, and repeating the process over again the next day. Sometimes I did that while vegging out on some Limited Edition Cookie Dough Oreos. With a mindset and feelings such as those, I needed help to keep me on point and motivated.

This is why I say—though I do not think the technology is required—if you are early in the process of losing weight, if you have fallen off the wagon, if you need something to add excitement to the process, if you need something to guide you, or if you need a push, then using technology is a great way to start you off and to get you back on track. Here is why, during the journey to losing seventy-five pounds, technology worked for me.

Counting Calories: What a Drag

I hate counting calories—hate it! In fact, I do not think you should have to count calories, but I understand now why it can be helpful. Counting, or least having an idea of the number of calories you are taking in, is instrumental in the weight-loss process. That is because, in order to lose weight, you need to take in fewer calories than you burn off. By tracking both your calories in and your calories out, you get a better sense of how you are progressing. How your clothes fit is also a great way to track how you are progressing (up or down), but, by knowing the amount of calories that you are taking in versus what you are putting out, you can make any necessary adjustments to both.

Back to me hating to count calories. I do not like to physically do it myself. Call me lazy or even high-maintenance (I am neither, for the record), but I simply have no desire to go through the process of reading a label, noting the food items, tracking the number of calories, and then adding them up for EVERY. SINGLE. THING. The simple thought of that exhausts me even as I write this.

Not only that, but it also made the idea of losing weight undesirable, no matter how necessary. But the thing was that I did want to and needed to lose weight. If I had to go through the laborious task just mentioned, I would have; however, during the journey of losing seventy-five pounds, I thankfully did not have to. My tools of the trade made that possible.

Make Knowing What You Eat Easy

Just as important as knowing your caloric intake are the ingredients in what you are eating. It is in your best interest to know the amount of carbohydrates, fat, protein, sugar, and sodium contained in your food. You can be taking in too much, or too little, of these nutrients and not realize it. Using these tools that I used will help you be better informed. Not only will you be better informed, but you also will get guidance on reading nutritional information labels, ingredients, and packaging headlines. I will go into packaging headlines deeper in "Chapter 7: Don't Be Fooled."

Until then, what you need to be conscious of is that some packaging headlines lead you to thinking you are choosing a healthy option, but, upon further inspection, that item you are considering is not the best for your weight-loss goal. That is why I am very diligent about reading nutritional information labels and ingredients.

Your Request is Granted

Ten years after my initial weight loss, some pretty bright people developed some rather amazing tools to help make calorie counting and tracking of carbohydrates, fat, protein, sodium and sugar a whole lot less labor-intensive. The technology is also pretty cool and eye-opening.

The technologies I will share with you offer what is important to me. They all are intuitive, require only a few steps, are portable, and are easy to use. All the heavy lifting is done for you. I will not hold out on you. Yes, sometimes a little extra work is required, but that little extra work is not off-putting. In fact, that little extra effort is quite cool.

To help me with the process of effortlessly tracking calories, carbohydrates, protein, fat, sugar, sodium, nutritional information, and ingredients, I use two pieces of technology: MyFitnessPal and Fooducate. Both work in the cloud, which means you can access them from the Internet or from a mobile device. Since my phone is practically glued to my hip, I access both tools from my iPhone 6 (as of the writing of this book). I could access them from my preferred web browser, but I connect through the dedicated applications. Here is how I use them.

HOW TO DO IT

Sign up for MyFitnessPal and Fooducate on the web. Do not worry: Both tools are FREE. Each does have a premium, or pro, version, requiring a monthly or annual payment. For my initial purposes, the free versions were all that I needed. All you will need to do is provide your email address and create a username and password. Then you can start using the tools.

MyFitnessPal About three months into the seventy-five-pound weight-loss journey, I started using MyFitnessPal to track my calorie intake and other nutritional information, such as carbohydrate, protein, sugar, sodium, and fat intake.

I am going to be straight up with you, as I have been and will do throughout this book. I used MyFitnessPal consistently during the first few months of my weight-loss journey. When I got to the point of eliminating certain foods from my diet and having a greater sense of what to eat for a healthier me, I stopped using it.

If I went through periods of about two to three weeks of not losing weight or gaining a couple of pounds, I would go back to MyFitnessPal to help me figure out what I might be consuming to cause that to happen. Usually, I found that, even though I thought I was eating fine, it turned out not to be the case. For example, I once got hooked on lattes from Starbucks and Dunkin' Donuts. At Starbucks, I would have it made with soy milk. At Dunkin' Donuts, I would order the Latte Lite, having it made with almond milk. Having those without sugar or without adding flavors, I thought I was doing great.

Here was the issue: I was having about two of those every day. When I started tracking those lattes in MyFitnessPal, my eyes were opened. With the help of MyFitnessPal, I realized I was consuming a lot of sugar from the soy milk and almond milk, especially due to the frequency and amount.

A bit puzzled by the amount of sugar in the almond milk, on one of my visits to Dunkin' Donuts, I took a peek at what kind of almond milk they were using. It was vanilla-flavored almond milk by Silk. One serving, which is one cup, contains ninety calories and sixteen grams of sugar. That was a huge difference between what I used at home and assumed, wrongfully so, that was also used by Dunkin'. At home, I sometimes used (still do) the Silk Original Unsweetened variety, which has thirty calories and zero grams of sugar.

So, I cut back on the lattes. The following week, the scale moved down two pounds. Knowing what I was putting into my body, because of MyFitnessPal and because I was paying attention to nutritional information (see "Chapter 7: Don't Be Fooled"), made that possible.

My suggestion to you is to count calories if and when you need to in order to keep you on track or get you back on track. As long as you are consuming wholesome, nutrient-rich foods regularly, calorie counting is not necessary. You can even eat a not-so-healthy treat in moderation (see more about treats and moderation in "Chapter 10: Tips, Tricks, and *Oh No I Won't*").

Conversely, if you are not yet to the point where you are knowledgeable or disciplined enough to do that on your own, use MyFitnessPal and Fooducate—I will discuss that in a little bit—to assist you until you can manage on your own. If you find yourself slipping, go back to using these tools to help you understand where you are faltering and to help you get back on track.

How to work MyFitnessPal

1. **Set up profile information and goals.** Besides not having a desire to count calories on my own, I also struggled with knowing how many calories to consume. I knew from my reading that we need our calorie intake to be less than our total daily calories burned, but what does that mean? In "Chapter 11: Move Your Body!" I will talk about workout DVDs that I use. Along with those DVDs, we receive meal planners, which include calorie calculations. The thing is, for some of them (P90X3, in particular), I was convinced I must have done the calculations incorrectly. There was no way in the world I could eat as much food, just for breakfast, that the calorie counter was suggesting. I found from reading forums that many people were in agreement with me. I eventually turned to MyFitnessPal for help. Go to Goals (on iPhone) or Settings (online), and then click on Update Your Diet Profile. Enter the parameters, such as your current weight, goal weight, and height, and select from the options for your weekly goal: pounds to lose, maintenance weight, and pounds to gain (yes, some people want or need to gain weight). What is great about MyFitnessPal is that it will not allow you to go under or over the safe level of weight loss or weight gain. That means if you desire to lose five pounds in a week, it will not allow you to select above two pounds, which is the maximum one should safely lose per week. You will also need to provide your gender and birthday (to calculate your age), select an option to describe your normal daily activities, select the number of workouts (from 0-7) that you perform per

week, enter the number of minutes you work out, and select how you want to track expended energy (in calories or in kilojoules). Based on those inputs, MyFitnessPal will estimate how many calories/kilojoules you need to consume for the day.

2. **Integrate tracking devices and digital scales.** If you have an application to track your specific activities or your activity throughout the day or a digital scale, check to see if MyFitnessPal will integrate with yours. On the MyFitnessPal menu, under Apps, is a list of applications that integrate with MyFitnessPal. If your app is not available, they are constantly adding devices; therefore, be sure to check back to see if your device has been included. As an alternative, you can download one of the available applications. I, for example, use Digifit to track the types of workouts I do. That includes running, INSANITY, INSANITY MAX:30, and my HIIT workout sessions with my personal trainer. It also tracks the number of calories, what percentage of those calories burned came from carbs, and what percentage came from fat. If you are a runner, it tracks your mileage, route run, and pace. To track my activity, such as steps taken, calories expended, and sleep activity, I wear a Misfit watch. It has become quite the conversation piece. You may be more familiar with the Fitbit. The Misfit does the same thing. I like it over the Fitbit because the Misfit is more versatile and handsome looking. Lastly, I integrate MyFitnessPal with my Withings Scale. It is a digital scale that tracks my weight, body fat (I am not all that convinced that it does a good job of this), and heart rate. These devices, working in combination with MyFitnessPal, allow it to track my calories out. It also helps MyFitnessPal to automatically adjust my weight and to track how many total calories I have available to consume during the day.

3. **Input everything you eat every day.** At first, this seems a bit much, but it gets to be a fun task over time. Also, it can be very eye-opening. I, for example, was astonished one day to see how many grams of sugar I was

consuming from a Dunkin' Donuts Latte Lite, even with almond milk and no added sugar. You will be surprised that, even if you think you are doing well with your choices, there are ingredients that can make it be otherwise. Over time, you will be surprised how astute you have become about what foods are best for you and how much you do not miss some of the foods that caused you to gain weight.

4. **Add your recipes to MyFitnessPal.** Earlier in the book, I mentioned that there is a little effort involved with these tools. When I stated that, I was referring to the adding of recipes. The really cool thing is that, if you have a recipe from the Internet, you can enter its URL, and MyFitnessPal will bring in each ingredient, the serving size, and the amount of each ingredient. The downside is that the process is not always perfect. Therefore, in some instances, you may be required to clean up the information. The great thing is that you only need to do it once for each recipe. It also gets to be a little more work if you modify recipes, like I do. In "Chapter 3: Get That C.R.A.P Out of My House," I discussed modifying foods that you really like but are fattening or loaded with sugar. When I find a recipe that falls into this category, after uploading it from the Internet, I then manually update the ingredient I plan to use instead.

5. **Read the blog posts.** Soon after you sign up with MyFitnessPal, you will start receiving emails from them in your inbox. In those emails, you will get information recommending exercises, success stories of people much like you, recipes, and any other bits of information to aid you in the weight-loss and weight-maintenance process.

Fooducate. I really like this tool. It provides a wealth of information. I like that it helps take out the guesswork. It helps you to be a more informed consumer of the foods that you are putting into your body. It helps open your eyes to what you may have considered as healthy but come to realize that it is indeed quite the opposite. You learn to not simply read what the front of the packaging tells you, but focus on what the nutritional information and ingredients tell you. Lastly, it will teach you to eat more natural foods than those that come in a box.

Here, I share how I use Fooducate. It has a health tracker, which is similar to how MyFitnessPal works, but I have yet to give that feature a try. The same goes for using the Fooducate community, Healthy Recipes (I will check that feature out, because I am always in need of a recipe since I am not creative enough to come up with my own), and a Daily Tip. The feature I use, almost exclusively (obviously), is the Food Finder. I use the Food Finder to prepare for a trip to the grocery store or while I am grocery shopping or at a store that sells on-the-go, packaged items. I particularly use it if I find an item intriguing but that makes me do a side-eye (is this really healthy?). I will speak more on that in Chapter 7 when I talk about not letting labels fool you.

How to use Fooducate

1. **Always have your mobile device when going food shopping.** My phone is always with me. That makes this application handy.

2. **Pick a food item and open the Fooducate application.** I take a food item, flip it to the barcode, open up my phone to the Fooducate app, and then open up Food Finder, which opens up a clear box. That is the device that reads the barcode of the food item. Point that box at the barcode.

3. **Review the product information.** Voila! Information about that item returns, provided that the food item is in the Fooducate database (there are many items in there).

4. **Review Product tab.** At the time of this writing, you will first be presented with the product page, which displays a letter grade, whether or not the food item is non-GMO, the number of calories per serving, and comments from people who have tried the item. There are also three

additional tabs: Explanations, Nutrition, and Alternatives. I'll break those down for you next.

5. **Review Explanations tab.** This tab gives you information, such as GMO probability, warnings about salt and sugar levels, and Food Points for people who use Weight Watchers, just to name a few sources of explanations. Any additional explanation is based on the type of food. For English muffins, for example, the Explanations section lets you know if the they contain whole grains (that is what you want to see) as an ingredient. Conversely, vitamin water will show recommendations stating, "Get your vitamins from real food," and advisories regarding the mention of natural flavors being added.

6. **Review Nutrition tab.** This tab displays the nutritional information about the product. MyFitnessPal provides this information as well, but Fooducate takes it a little further with what it provides. Fooducate gives focus to the areas you should care about, such as fat, cholesterol, sodium, and sugar. If any of these is deemed especially good, a green check mark is displayed. In the case of that vitamin water I mentioned, a red check mark appears next to sugars. (Just so that you know, the flavor of vitamin water I researched also had a grade of *C+*.) This page also includes the ingredients and a link to report if any of this information is incorrect. That, I think, is pretty awesome.

7. **Review Alternatives tab.** It is my practice to review the Alternatives tab after skimming the Product tab. This is especially the case if the product is rated poorly. In my case, *poorly* is anything less than an *A*, but realistically it is anything less than a *B*. This is an awesome part of the tool. It will display, as the name suggests, alternatives to the item you choose. Provided is the name of the alternative product, a photo of the item (sometimes the current packaging looks a little different), the letter grade assigned to the product, calories per serving, and mention of whether the product is a Top Product, non-GMO, or GMO.

8. **Decide whether or not to put the product in your basket.** Didn't I tell you that Fooducate provides you with a wealth of information? With it, you get better at making informed decisions. I always aim to choose products with a grade of an *A*, but that is not always possible. Therefore, I am usually happy with a grade of a *B*. I only choose a grade of a *C+* or *C* if a recipe calls for something that I cannot produce myself and the alternatives have the same grade. When that happens, I then look for what is the least offensive in terms of non-GMO versus GMO, meaning I will go with a GMO item if the other nutritional information is not too damaging. My thinking is that the product is not a main source of the recipe, so that little bit is not going to hurt. Those are the decisions you will be making too.

9. **Read the Pro Tips.** There is a lot of research about what to eat and what not to eat. I mentioned in the beginning that it all can get quite confusing after a while. Also, doing research on your own can be time-consuming, though I believe it is prudent on our parts. Even so, Fooducate uses Pro Tips to share research with you by email. You can also access them from your Fooducate account. I read them from the Fooducate app on my iPhone. I call it the "I was wondering about that" section. For example, there was one article called, "Is a Low-Carb Diet Right for You?" Like with all articles, the information is shared in a very easy-to-read, not-too-technical way. Each article also ends with the "Bottom Line" summary. As with anything, it is up to you to decide what you will do with the information. I am sharing it because I find it informative and relatable.

Keeping-It-Real Solutions and Helpful Tips for Your Struggles, Challenges, and Excuses

You don't own a smartphone or tablet. Yes, without a smartphone or tablet you will not have the conveniences of tracking information immediately; however, you can use a desktop computer to update your information. This is because both of these tools are accessible from the Internet. Go to myfitnesspal.com for MyFitnessPal and fooducate.com for Fooducate to update the information.

Regarding Fooducate, you will have to plan ahead before grocery shopping. That is something you should be doing anyway. You know this from what you learned in the first four chapters. There will be more on grocery shopping in the next chapter. I use Fooducate at the grocery store for items I did not verify before going shopping, because I am buying an item I was not intending to purchase, or out of curiosity about nutritional information and ingredients.

You don't own a personal desktop. I am not trying to be funny or facetious here. For some families, it is their reality to not own computers. In such cases, I recommend going to your public library, as most public libraries today have computers. Reaching out to family members or friends who are willing to be accountability partners is also an option.

1. **Schedule time to go to the library or to meet with your family member or friend**: You know your schedule. Verify the hours for your public library; then determine the days and times you will go to the library. If working with a reliable family member or friend, set a day and time you will always get together to update your information. You must schedule this time. If you do not, you are less likely to commit to making these updates.

2. **Jot down in a notebook each of your meals**: You will have to be more diligent about jotting down on paper what you have eaten, but you can make this work.

3. **Go to the library, family member, or friend to update your information, to look up information, or for planning time**: Use your time at the library or with the person letting you use their devices to update MyFitnessPal with your meals. You can also use this time to look

up information about what you are planning to purchase in both MyFitnessPal and Fooducate. Use this as your planning time. As you make your grocery list, for example, you can use Fooducate to look up the best item for what you want to buy. Note: you will be at a slight disadvantage because not every grocery store sells the same brands. Therefore, something that you see as an option on Fooducate may not be at your grocery store. I have a suggestion for that too. As my oldest nephew, who is seven at the time of this writing, says, "I have a solution." See the next point.

4. **Bring a friend or family member with a smartphone or tablet grocery shopping with you**: See, I told you I had a solution. When you are committed to being a healthier, better you, your brain works to find a way. With your friend, you can use Fooducate to help you get additional information about a food item.

You do not want to do any of this tracking stuff. Hey, I do not blame you. It can be cumbersome. Tracking what you eat and verifying what is in your food is merely a recommendation. I found that it was useful to me to set a foundation and become more knowledgeable and informed. If you do not want to track anything or look anything up, that is your decision. However, I do recommend that, if you do not track what you are eating or do not do your due diligence before buying certain foods, you at least reference my website, pamelaburke.com/dietfreeme-resources, for a list a recommended foods. After trying that, if you find you are still struggling to lose weight, I recommend that you come back to this chapter and implement using these tools.

You Have the Tools: Get Ready to Be a Master Shopper

Though it is recommended, not necessary, to count your calories or know every detail about what you eat, you at least know you have tools at your disposal if you should ever need them. By using MyFitnessPal, you can track your caloric intake and other important nutritional information, get a gage of how you are progressing, and make informative adjustments, if necessary. With Fooducate, you can research nutritional information, ingredients, and the health-and-wellness factor of a product before you buy it. In the next chapter, we will discuss your grocery-shopping strategy. I will keep repeating this: Your weight loss for life success is dependent upon planning and preparation. Let's go plan for grocery shopping.

Your grocery cart
tells your story.
Make sure yours
tells how much
you love a healthy you.

CHAPTER 6

FROM GROCERY-SHOPPING FLUNKY TO MASTER SHOPPER

At this point, it should be clear to you how much the role of planning and preparation plays in helping you lose weight and keep it off. Thus far, every chapter has touched on planning and preparation in some form. Your mind is in a different space, as you know how vital it is to be mentally prepared for your weight-loss success. You are clear about changing your relationship with food and using technology, such as MyFitnessPal and Fooducate, to help you become an informed consumer of what you eat. In this chapter, we expand upon the last by entering the grocery store. As we lead into this chapter, I will share with you how I feel about grocery shopping and my history with it before losing weight.

Grocery Shopping Was Fun as a Kid

Do you recall how I felt about counting calories? If not, shoot back to Chapter 5. I used some strong language in saying that I hate it. Right up there with it is grocery shopping. It's odd, because, as a kid, I looked forward to going grocery shopping with my mother, especially on double-coupon days.

That was my opportunity to feel like an adult. Mom would collect all of her coupons, and then, on double-coupon day, she would give me a list of groceries to get while she tended to her list.

I recall proudly walking the aisles, collecting my items, meeting up with my mother at the designated meet-up place in the grocery store, and then proceeding to the register with my coupons in hand, along with the money my mother had given me to pay for the groceries. I have no idea with my adult mind why I found that so much fun, but, at this stage in my life, I do not find it fun at all.

When it comes to grocery shopping, I am nowhere near as prudent with knowing the sales on groceries like my mother did (and still does today). Coupon clipping? Bah! Good luck with that. As someone who likes to think of herself as frugal, one might think I would give coupon clipping more attention. But, more than anything, I dread grocery shopping.

Anything but Grocery Shopping—PLEASE!!

A typical grocery-shopping day for me includes getting the bare essentials: milk (in my case, almond milk), eggs, water, and toilet paper. When I am on my best behavior and need to go, I still despise it, because I do not like the crowds. As a kid, that did not bother me. As an adult, I have to work hard to be strategic about when I go.

I usually cannot go when I want to go. I wake up before most grocery stores open. If I go when the doors open, they are restocking the shelves. Often that means what I want has not been restocked yet. Then, waiting until a time when the peak hours have died down means the shelves are practically bare again.

Using the services of the grocery store or someone else to shop for me is an option, but I am a bit finicky about who handles my things. Besides, I do not get to play with my Fooducate app if someone else does the grocery shopping for me.

Cry All You Want; Grocery Shopping Is a Necessity

No matter how I feel about the grocery-shopping process, it needs to get done. Not only that, but it also needs to get done in a way that helps me maintain my weight loss and in a way for you to do the same or lose weight. In order to do that, I implemented a strategy to make sure that happens.

HOW TO DO IT

Eat first. Go grocery shopping after eating. You will be less likely to put in your basket what you should not be eating. Think about it. Have you ever gone grocery shopping while hungry? Did you find yourself buying everything under the sun, especially foods that you know are not going to be kind to your waistline? Whether you have had this experience or not, trust me: Eat a healthy and filling meal before you head to the grocery store.

Drink water. Drinking water is a great way to fill up without unwanted calories. It's the same concept as eating before going grocery shopping.

Avoid aisle shopping. Aisle shopping is when you walk up and down each aisle, coming up with your grocery list as you go. You walk the aisle, see an item, and say, "Oh yes, I need that." That method of shopping is not an issue until you hit the aisle with soda, juice, cookies, and chips. Those aisles are loaded with sugary, high-calorie, overly processed foods that offer no nutritional value. Not only that, if you shop those aisles, you may be tempted to get something you should not have.

Not even after losing weight did I shop those aisles. Yes, now I walk down them, but I can do that without an issue, because those foods are not a part of my lifestyle. I suggest, unless you are getting water, which is usually at the end of the soda aisle, until you also get to the place where those foods are not a part of your lifestyle, that you be certain to skip those aisles. The next two grocery-shopping suggestions help you stay away from the soda, cookies, and ice cream aisles.

67

Prepare a list. Like with eating first, having a list of what you need before you get to the grocery store will help you refrain from the not-so-healthy stuff. Your list is your focus. If, however, you recall a food item that was not on your list, make sure it is something wholesome. Forgetting the Oreos or Lay's potato chips is a good thing. Leave them on the shelf. Likewise, if there is an item that was on your list and you are not too sure it falls into the good-for-you category, bust out your Fooducate app to help you. Refer to the previous chapter for further information on Fooducate.

Shop the perimeter. Spend more time shopping the perimeter. This is where fresh items, such as produce, meat, and seafood will be found. I am only familiar with grocery stores in the United States. What I can tell you with almost 100-percent certainty is that they are all set up the same. These items are on the outer perimeter of the grocery store. If you need to move inward, let it be for cleansers, greeting cards, and condiments that you do not make for yourself.

Do not shop by food labels. I do not want to go into this topic too much here because I will go into detail about it in the next chapter. I will say this: You will run into instances where you see a label that states "low-fat." Do not buy that item just because it is being promoted as low-fat. Be an informed consumer. Use an app, such as Fooducate. That will give you a sense of how processed that item is, or not. It will also let you know if what you are really about to purchase is something perhaps low in fat but high in sugar.

Keeping-It-Real Solutions and Helpful Tips for Your Struggles, Challenges, and Excuses

I do not like grocery shopping. Did you see the opening to this chapter? I don't like it either. In order to survive, we need to eat. We must get our groceries somehow. Shop for your food online. Many grocery stores today offer that option. You then have the choice, in most cases, to have the food delivered or pick it up yourself at the store. I personally have only done this once. That is only because I have control issues and because I messed up my order. When it came to picking fruit, I thought the quantity of one meant one pound. Ha ha ha...silly me. It actually meant exactly what was in my bag when we picked up the groceries from the store: one apple, one pear, one orange, and one banana. (Should I be embarrassed to have admitted that?) I know better now but have yet to try that again. Give it try. It is a great alternative. Just remember when getting fruit that the quantity of one means exactly that.

I am too busy to go grocery shopping. I have a lot on my plate too. I work a full-time job; I write for my blog, canwilldone.com; I am writing this book; I want to make sure I do not take my spouse for granted; and, as of the writing of this chapter, I am in the process of packing to move to a new home. I truly understand busy.

As I had to tell myself a time or two, if this was something you really wanted to do, you would make time to do it. Here is something I know too: If you do not make the time for grocery shopping, you must count on yourself being disciplined enough to make the right choices when eating out.

If you are currently not in the space where you are disciplined enough to do that, then choose the frequency (weekly, biweekly) and time you will go grocery shopping. As I have had to adjust my schedule to make time to write this book, it has become clearer how important it is to specify where, when, and what time.

I have kids; they will want all the foods I am trying not to eat. How you raise your kids and run your home is your business. I cannot and will not tell you what to do in terms of raising your children. I will let you know that I understand. I have nieces and nephews. Given the choice between eating vegetables or sugary snacks, they are going to choose the sugary snacks every single time.

The thing is, when they are with Aunt Pam (that's me) there are no sugary or fattening treats to be had at my house. This is not to instill deprivation. I do that for me. I know if I were to keep a bag of Chips Ahoy! cookies in my house, there is a chance that having one cookie would turn into devouring a lot of cookies. While that type of food is not in my home, I do not miss it. Not only that, when I am away from home, I do not miss it either. Since the food is not in my home, the kids are not expecting it. That is what I am encouraging you to do. Like I mentioned earlier in "Chapter 3: Get That C.R.A.P Out of My House," if you do not make those types of foods available in your home, there is no expectation to have them.

Do Not Get It Twisted

I most definitely allow myself to have a cookie, some of a slice of apple pie with vanilla ice cream on top, an occasional sugared raised donut from Dunkin' Donuts, or even a cupcake. I do not consider it a treat or a cheat item (see more about "cheating" in "Chapter 10: Tips, Tricks, and *Oh No I Won't* "). I consider it something I wanted; therefore, I had it. On those rare occasions that I go that route, moderation is always the intention. It also helps that I kick my behind most days of the week with exercise. It is not "exercise so I can eat whatever I want." It is "exercise to exercise the practice of living a healthy lifestyle."

The bottom line is that I have no intention of depriving myself, nor will I suggest that you feel deprived. I only suggest that you be mindful and informed of what you are doing for your health and your body. When you follow what I prescribe throughout this book, you will find that you are not in danger of risking your hard work or of falling completely off the wagon.

Protection from Lack of Honesty

Speaking of not being mindful and informed, and risking your hard work, we need to have a critical eye when it comes to food labels. On my Twitter feed, twitter.com/canwilldone, one of my posts resulted in being followed by an email and content marketer. Taking a look at her posts, one in particular caught my eye. The headline was, "If Big Name Companies Were More 'Honest' With Their Branding." A corresponding image appeared: the McDonald's logo with the tagline, "Makes You Fat." That tagline reminded me of food labels, if they were to be honest. It is for this reason that we have the next chapter. We do not want dishonest labels to fool us into becoming unhealthy or increasing our waistlines.

Show food-branding
companies you're not
fooled by their lies.

CHAPTER 7

DON'T BE FOOLED

Here we are at Chapter 7, about to start the second half of the book, and guess what: The contents of this chapter, like those preceding it, are still about planning and preparation. Yes, planning and preparation are that serious. If you want the benefit of being more confident (I sure hope you do), if you want the benefit of being prepared for life's challenges, and if you want the benefit of enjoying weight loss for a lifetime, I cannot stress enough how important planning and preparation are to your ability in achieving that. By not being fooled by label wordsmithing, you will be enhancing those benefits.

You Know It's Not Healthy, but the Words Suggest Otherwise

In "Chapter 4: Don't Be Caught with Your Pants Down—Be Prepared," when talking about planning and being prepared, I mentioned that I would visit the vending machine between classes while I was in graduate school, during which time I went from being healthy to eating whatever, and that whatever was far from what could be considered healthy.

I did at least try to make smart decisions, or so I thought. I recall standing in front of the machine, perusing the contents in something that would be evidence of trying to make wise choices. As my eyes scanned, skipping over one item after another, I would come upon a 1.125-ounce single-serve bag of Baked Lay's. That seemed promising. I thought baked was much better for me than fried. It also helped that my portion would be controlled if I stuck to one of those small bags. OK, so Baked Lay's looked like a good option, but sometimes I craved something sweet and kept looking. That is when I would stop at a package of 2.5-ounce strawberry Twizzler twists. What was it that caught my eye? Well, I was always a fan of those, but what made them seem OK was the label on the front of the package: low-fat. Even though I knew it was a candy, low-fat psychologically said to me that it was alright to satisfy my sweet craving, because, hey, it was low-fat.

Have you done that—based your decision to purchase a food product based on the label that was screaming at you, "Hey You!! Yes, you know that candy is not a healthy option, but I am low-fat, so that makes me OK!! You know you want me"? The next thing you know, you are enjoying your treat that promises low-fat, so you are not adding *that* much fat to your diet. Granted, if you have some idea of what foods are considered healthy and which ones are not, you know that chips and candy are not going to be anywhere near the top of the healthy-item list. Heck, they should not be on the list at all. I use them as examples, because these are the types of foods we crave.

The Label Says It's Alright to Have It

We especially crave them in those times or situations in our lives that I mentioned in "Chapter 2: When You Have Had Enough, Dig Deep into Your *Why?*" It is when you are at your most vulnerable, due to stress, lack of sleep, sadness, and uncertainty, that you will seek out such foods.

Even if you are consciously adhering to a healthy lifestyle, in your moments of despair, if you are craving such foods as chips and candy, your mind is fooled into having the chips and candy, because that label says it is alright to have it.

In this chapter, I am here to tell you not to be fooled by food labels. They are misleading. They are meant to have you go through that dialog I went through above. We are going to make wiser decisions by ignoring what the front label says in favor of what it says on the back of the label.

HOW TO DO IT

Flip to the ingredients. Skip what it says on the front of the package. Go immediately to the ingredients. Packages vary, but most items have the ingredients on the back. If the ingredients are not on the back, you will find them on the side.

Understand how ingredients work. When ingredients are listed on food packages, they are listed differently than recipe ingredients. On recipes, ingredients are typically listed in the order in which they are used in the recipe. On food packages, the ingredients are listed in order of the main ingredient, meaning from the most prominent ingredient to the least prominent ingredient. Let's use the Baked Lay's and Twizzlers as examples.

The first five ingredients in Baked Lay's are dried potatoes, corn starch, sugar, corn oil, and salt. For Twizzlers, the "low-fat" candy, the first ingredients are corn syrup and enriched wheat, which itself has several ingredients. Of those, the only ones most of us are familiar with are flour, sugar, and cornstarch. I am not even going to add the fifth item because I have no idea what it is. It is just hints of a bunch of other stuff—seriously, I mean *stuff*. Go get a package to see for yourself.

Scrutinize the ingredients.
Baked Lay's

Potatoes are packed with nutritional and weight-conscious benefits. They are a nutrient-dense food, which means they offer a lot of nutrients but have relatively few calories. They are fibrous and high in potassium, which is great in relation to reducing blood pressure. That is all great as long as you are sure not to fry them. But these are baked, not fried. Let's keeping digging by breaking down the next two ingredients.

Corn starch: Recall I mentioned that potatoes are a nutrient-dense food? Well, corn starch does not have one iota of nutritional value. All corn starch offers is additional calories. We have already established that, in order to lose weight, you want to reduce calories. To maintain your weight, you do not want to take in too many calories, and you most certainly do not want to take in calories that offer no nutritional benefit.

Sugar: Fructose is highly prevalent in sugar. Fructose is not essential for our bodies to function. When we take in too much of this nonessential product, that fructose turns to fat. Sugar also offers no nutritional value as it has no vitamins or minerals. Once again, those Baked Lay's have an ingredient that contains empty calories by using sugar.

In my family, it is not uncommon to hear someone utter the phrase, "You know she has sugar." That is another way of referencing that someone is insulin-dependent because they have type II diabetes. This happens because sugar causes a resistance to insulin. The fact that sugar is the third ingredient should be an immediate turnoff.

The bottom line is keep the Baked Lay's in the vending machine or on the shelf.

Twizzlers

Corn syrup: Corn syrup is 100-percent glucose, which is sugar. We already covered sugar in breaking down the ingredients of Baked Lay's.

I am not going to bother going into the remaining ingredients. It does not matter that Twizzlers are low-fat (four pieces are 0.5 grams of fat, according to the packaging). I am stopping here because the number-one ingredient is sugar.

Do you now see why it is so important to skip the labeling on the front of foods and why you need to read the ingredients?

Do your homework and stay informed. OK, I admit that it is a bit of a pain in the butt to set aside time to do research, but that time is well worth it when it comes to your health and well-being. Some of the information I shared with you above is common knowledge, but it is surface knowledge. For instance, we know that sugar is not the best for us, but it is important that we understand *why* it is not the best for us. By doing your homework instead of simply saying to yourself, "I am not going to have this, because it is all sugar," you would say, "The fructose from sugar is what causes fat; that is why I am not going to have it." See how the latter holds so much more meaning? That is why you need to do your homework. At pamelaburke.com/dietfreeme-resources, I provide you with some common labels that should cause you pause. What I share with you is what you should be mindful of checking.

No doubt, it is extremely difficult to stay on top of all the latest studies. Most of us are not nutritionists, dietitians, or health professionals. With that being the case, it is not our life's work to stay abreast of all the information that is available. At a minimum, I use the tools that were referenced in "Chapter 5: Tools of the Trade—the Go-To Technology," to assist me with being an informed consumer of foods that are good for my body, mind, and health. When I really want to know something, I take the time to do a little extra digging. Google is my go-to source. I highly recommend that you too use these methods to help keep you informed. And, as I have said throughout this book, listen to your body. Foods that are not good for one person may be perfectly fine for you. So, that person recommending that you go gluten-free has good intentions, but you may very well be able to handle gluten just fine. Pay attention to what your body tells you, and you will know for sure.

Keeping-It-Real Solutions and Helpful Tips for Your Struggles, Challenges, and Excuses

The labels can't lie. Labels may not lie, but they most certainly can mislead. Take a look at what I provided above about the breakdown of Twizzlers. The front of the package has "low-fat" in yellow to help the words stick out. When you flip to the nutritional information, next to fat you will indeed see zero grams. That makes the label true. What makes it misleading is the effects of its core ingredient: sugar. The fructose from the sugar adds unwanted fat to your body.

I want to have a treat sometimes, no matter what the label says. So do I. That is why I will indulge. The key is the frequency of your indulgence. Having a package of Twizzlers, or the like, every once in a blue moon is not a deal breaker. Also know that too much of anything, no matter how healthy it is for you, will cause you to gain weight. The key to this section of the book is to be mindful and not let labels lead you astray to the point that you eat it, especially more of it, because the label makes you believe it is better for you.

There is too much information to know. Make life easy for yourself. If you do not know, do not have it, or do not have much of it. Another option is to use applications such as Fooducate, which was mentioned in "Chapter 5: Tools of the Trade—the Go-To Technology." The app helps take the guesswork out, thus making life easier.

Knowledge is Empowering

Did that knowledge I dropped on you seem impressive? What I shared with you just now, both the facts about ingredients and how to avoid being fooled by label wordsmithing, I learned by doing exactly what I recommended to you: research. When I do not know something, when something does not seem quite right, or when I want to better informed, I do research. There is nothing more detrimental and demoralizing than ignorance. You counteract that ignorance with knowledge. The saying goes, "Knowledge is power." I believe that knowledge is empowering. Empower yourself. Start flipping to the ingredients, scrutinizing ingredients, and learning about key ingredients. Use tools like Fooducate to make your life easier. Having soaked up this knowledge, do your body good by adding water to your life. That is where we are heading now with the next chapter.

If you are only drinking water to quench your thirst, you are missing out on goodness.

CHAPTER 8

WATER DOES A BODY
AND MIND GOOD

At this point, you are super-focused. You understand why you reach for foods that expand your waistline, and you now have strategies to save you from yourself. You have mental tools, and you have physical and digital tools to assist you. In this chapter, we focus on what none of us can do without in order to survive: water. I know that water has been a great source for feeding my mind and body. Here, I show you how water has assisted me, before diving into how you can use water to do the same.

A Sistah Ain't Got Time for Water Breaks

Water is one of those things that I knew was good for me. At a high level, I knew that eight glasses of water a day were recommended. My problem was that I never took time to make sure I had enough of it. For me, getting my work done for my job and school was more important than stopping for water refills. My only exception was if—and that was a big IF—I had managed to get in a workout. That was about the only guarantee that I would get some water.

81

While taking computer courses and in graduate school, working out was highly unlikely; hence, along with all my bad eating habits, I gained so much weight. In fact, being sure to drink water was nowhere in the front of my mind. Other than the "once in a blue moon" workout and coincidental water-based food, the only time I purposefully sought out water was when I was thirsty. Apparently, I was not thirsty nearly enough.

Ah, So That's Why We Should Drink Water

That was unfortunate, because, when I finally got my mind in place to start taking better care of myself, water became one of my key success factors. You see, by me drinking water, I did not find myself eating even when I was not hungry. In fact, I felt full, which helped me not to eat too much. Eating in moderation was something I could do without trying.

When I made those unwanted trips to the grocery store, I was not drawn to foods I should not have. Why? Because I went to the grocery store full. Sometimes it was because of what I mentioned in "Chapter 6: From Grocery-Shopping Flunky to Master Shopper": I was full from eating before going shopping. But, more often than not, it was because of another tip I shared in that same chapter: I was full from drinking water before going grocery shopping.

Another thing I noticed from my drinking water is that I had more energy. Water played a part in giving me a boost. Yes, I visited the restroom often, but, given the benefits, those trips were well worth it. That is why this chapter is dedicated to making sure you drink water. I will share with you a recommended daily amount of water as well as ways to get that recommended amount of water.

HOW TO DO IT

Know how much water to drink. The rule of thumb was to drink eight glasses of water, but I always ended up asking, "Eight glasses of what size—

eight ounces, twelve ounces, sixteen ounces?" On my journey to losing seventy-five pounds, my personal trainer gave me an "amount of water to drink" prescription that was easy to follow. That is the one I still prescribe to. Drink, in ounces, half your body weight in water. If, for instance, you weigh 200 pounds, then drink 100 ounces of water a day.

Optimal time to drink water. All types of times have been recommended to me for drinking and not drinking water. Drink water thirty minutes before eating. Don't drink water until at least an hour after eating. Don't drink water while you are eating. Drink water first thing in the morning. I cannot be caught up in all of that. It is another one of those areas where I suggest you do what works for your body, which you will learn with practice.

After reading *The 5 A.M. Miracle: Dominate Your Day Before Breakfast* by Jeff Sanders, I start most mornings with a liter of water. I have to use the bathroom several times before catching the bus to work, since there is no restroom on the bus, but the water wakes me up and hydrates me after a night's sleep.

During the day, I drink water before I eat, which, at my best, is five small meals a day. I will have that water anywhere between forty-five minutes to just before I eat. When eating out, I may have sips of water during dinner, but that's rare. I also tend not to drink water directly after dinner, because my stomach sometimes does not handle that well. I also stay hydrated during my workouts and runs over six miles, but I don't count that in my daily intake of water.

Keeping-It-Real Solutions and Helpful Tips for Your Struggles, Challenges, and Excuses

I do not like the way water tastes. Usually water does not have a taste, at least in my opinion. I have, however, had tap water that was less than pleasant. Here are some suggestions to make water taste better.

1. **Add natural flavor.** When I say natural flavors, I am referring to flavor from cut fruit. Cut up some fruit and add it to the water. You can get creative here with flavors. You can use one type of fruit or a mixture. Go wild. You can also add leafy items, such as mint, for flavoring. I am not a fan of mint, but an aunt once made a concoction with mint, strawberries, and cucumber. Had I not seen it, I would have had no clue that mint was added.

2. **Invest in a water diffuser.** When you are on the go, take a water diffuser along with you. In it you can add your fruit.

3. **Add water enhancers.** There's no time to cut up some fruit? Water enhancers are an option. Not all are good for you; some are loaded with artificial colors and sweeteners. This is when a tool such as Fooducate comes in handy. An example of good water-enhancer options are those by Great Value, Dasani, and Stur.

That is too much water; I cannot drink that much water. In this case, get your water from food. Examples of foods you can use to get water are watermelon, celery, cucumber, lettuce, and strawberries. What is cool about these foods is that they also provide other nutrients.

Water is More Than a Thirst-Quencher

Water is your weapon against eating too much and buying food you do not need. You saw that in Chapter 6. This chapter was dedicated to making the consumption of water a habit. We now leave this chapter to help you put everything you have learned thus far into a package. And this discussion of water comes up there and in the two chapters that follow. That's how beneficial water is to you. It's time to put all this knowledge together. On to Chapter 9.

You've got the knowledge,
which gives you power;
now put it all to good use.

PUTTING IT ALL TOGETHER

You know you need to be prepared in order to be successful on your journey toward losing weight and sustaining that weight loss. You have tools that you can use to make your life easier in figuring out what to eat and what not to eat. You have your shopping strategies. Lastly, from the prior chapter, you know to drink plenty of water in order to do your body and mind good. Being prepared, using helpful tools, and drinking plenty of water—what else could there be?

Before Knowing Better

In this chapter, I will show you how I put all of the previous information together to help get me where I am today: sitting here, proudly writing a book for you with more confidence than I had two years ago at this time.

While in the computer programming courses and graduate school, I made a lot of mistakes when it came to eating. As discussed in "Chapter 2: When You Have Had Enough, Dig Deep into Your *Why?*" I was not prepared for the life change. In not being prepared for the life change, I picked up unhealthy habits. I did not sleep enough. I ate too many unhealthy and fattening choices. Drinking an adequate amount of water, as prescribed in "Chapter 8: Water Does a Body, and Mind Good," was an afterthought—if I thought about it at all. Without having meals prepared beforehand, as discussed in "Chapter 4: Don't Be Caught with Your Pants Down—Be Prepared," I gravitated to junk foods, such as candy, pizza, and fried chicken. Even when I tried to be health-conscious during those years, I still was not on the right track. As discussed in "Chapter 7: Don't Be Fooled," I would fall victim to the food-label trap, thinking that foods labeled "low-fat" or "low-calorie" were healthy options. Living such a lifestyle, especially during graduate school, when I was ten years older with a much slower metabolism, proved to be more detrimental. That was evident in how much weight I gained during those four years.

When You Know Better, You Do Better

The good news is that, by using all I have shared with you thus far, my life changed. I am a more informed consumer of food. That includes the approach I take when grocery shopping, which was referenced in "Chapter 6: From Grocery-Shopping Flunky to Master Shopper," and using technology to help make the decision-making process easier, as mentioned in "Chapter 5: Tools of the Trade—The Go-To Technology."

In this chapter, I will share my approach to food consumption. I combined what I learned from reading *Body for Life* to lose fifty pounds in 2001, with tricks I came up with to help me be successful during my journey to losing seventy-five pounds and making certain to keep that weight off for life.

During the span in which I lost the seventy-five pounds, work colleagues presumed I was losing the weight by not eating. I was frequently asked this question in slightly different variations: "When are you going to start eating again?" After being asked those questions time and time again, in some form or another, I came to the conclusion that people believed I was living on salads, a diet full of restrictions, or what may very well be cardboard. The thing is that I never stopped eating, nor did I do anything close to what would resemble starvation. I most certainly did not eat cardboard-like food. Salads were not and still are not a staple in my diet; I eat them, but not that much. And, as hard as it is for people to believe, my diet is not super-restrictive.

HOW TO DO IT

Starvation is not an option: eat frequent small meals. If you too are under the presumption that your weight loss must be aided by darn near starving yourself, let this tip strike that thought out of the forefront of your mind for good: I aim for six small meals per day. Yes, six. Try as I might to eat six meals, I typically eat five small meals by the end of the day.

I have read disputes about the validity of eating five to six small meals. If you do searches, you will likely find the same. I believe you can find something to dispute just about everything. All I can tell you is that eating five to six small meals is what works for me. Doing so helps me control the amount of calories I take in each day. It also helps avoid the risk of eating too much at each meal if I were to only eat three times a day. With the combination of frequent meals and water consumption, as mentioned in Chapter 8, overeating and taking in too many calories is really hard to accomplish. I eat two snacks a day. One is between breakfast and lunch. The other is between lunch and dinner.

Make sure each meal has three parts. Every meal should consist of a protein, carbohydrate, and fat. I am not too strict about the percentage of each, but I do lean heavily on the protein side and get carbohydrates from vegetables. I am mindful of my carbohydrate intake from other sources. It may all be in my head, but I swear I gain five pounds just thinking about eating bread. Vegetables are a great option. They are low in calories but high in volume. As a result, you can eat more and feel fuller on fewer calories. So, if you like the feeling of eating, eat more vegetables. (Smile.) I share what a typical day looks like for me below.

Have snacks as part of your small meals. Even though I am calling them small meals, two of those "meals," as I stated above, are snacks. The snacks are pretty light. That simply means they consist of fewer calories than what I consume at breakfast, lunch, and dinner. How many calories? Oh heck, I do not know. Like I mentioned in Chapter 5, I do not aim for a number. If I did, I would probably drive myself nuts and would not have made it this far. Luckily, with technology such as MyFitnessPal, calories can be monitored, but I most certainly am not a slave to calorie counting. If, however, that is what you need to succeed, by all means, knock yourself out and count those calories. Snack suggestions are provided at pamelaburke.com/dietfreeme-resources.

Have your food baked, steamed, grilled, or raw. Baked, steamed, grilled, or raw are the methods for cooking, or not, my meals. Did you notice what type of preparation is excluded? That's right: fried. The closest I have to fried food is the occasional donut. At this point in my life, because of maintaining a healthy lifestyle, I can barely stand the smell of fried food, let alone eat it. I fear my stomach would go into shock and I would get ill.

Every once in a very blue moon, if I want some fried chicken, I will cook up a batch using Rocco Dispirito's Flash-Fried Finger-Lickin' Chicken Recipe. Ask one of my cousins, though, and he will tell you in no way is that fried chicken. In fact, he has gone as far as to tell me not to bring that to a family function ever again as a fried-chicken option. I have every intention of ignoring that particular request. You will learn to ignore such things too. You will see what I mean when you get to "Chapter 10: Tips, Tricks, and *Oh No I Won't.*"

Eat real food: fresh and natural foods instead of boxed food. Isn't all food real food? In a word, no.

I do my best to avoid processed food in favor of real food. That means, if it comes in a box or a package, I do my best to avoid it. What is real food?

I recall that, when doing my search for that answer, there was not just one answer. When taking all the definitions together, real food came down to meaning food that is minimally processed, leaving it close to its natural state. That begs the question, "Well, what does that mean?"

I used to think that meant, if it comes in a package, bag, or box, you should not eat it, but that line of thinking was not valid. Oatmeal, for example, comes in a package, but it's great for you if you get the right kind. Let me give you some information on the benefits of oatmeal; then I will continue on with real food.

Oatmeal is a well-balanced meal choice. It contains both soluble and insoluble fiber as well as protein. It provides important minerals and, like with vegetables, it makes you feel fuller longer. My brand of choice is Bob's Red Mill Organic Thick Rolled Oats. It has one ingredient: organic whole grain oats. It contains five grams of fiber, seven grams of protein, and one gram of sugar.

Here is the key: Once extras, such as sugar and artificial flavors, are added, that oatmeal is no longer a real food. That is why it is so important to read the ingredients for the foods that you eat. Do this exercise: If you eat or are considering the instant variety of oatmeal (in the package, with fruit and flavoring already added), compare the nutritional information of that packet with the brand I eat. Enough said.

A simple rule of thumb is that, if the ingredients include preservatives, additives, colorings, artificial flavors, sweeteners, and chemicals (that stuff you can barely pronounce), you should avoid it.

Using an application like Fooducate also makes this a lot easier for you to discern what level of processing a food is—or rather, how real it is not.

Opt for eating veggies. Imagine a plate. Divide that plate in half with an imaginary line. On one half of that plate, add green fresh vegetables. Organic would be great, but it is not necessary.

Eat fruit. Select fruits that do not come in a can. Eat an orange, apple, pear, or grapes for a mid-morning or mid-afternoon snack. Add frozen fruits, like berries, peaches, bananas, and mangoes, to smoothies.

Cut the white stuff: salt and sugar. Put the salt shaker away. Use Mrs. Dash instead. There are a variety for you to try. We touched on this in "Chapter 3: Get That C.R.A.P. Out of My House," but, as a reminder, cut back on or eliminate soda, fruit juices (even if the bottle says 100-percent natural), and energy drinks. Refrain from adding sugar to beverages. Do not use artificial sweeteners, such as Splenda or Sweet'N Low, in its place.

Replace refined carbohydrates. Replace white pasta, white rice, and foods made with white flour, such as crackers and pretzels, with whole grain carbohydrates, such as whole wheat breads, pastas, bulgur, oatmeal, quinoa, and brown rice.

Remember "Chapter 7: Don't Be Fooled"? This is a great time to be well-informed. Which do you think is the most beneficial, multigrain or whole grain? I know that, before I did some research, I believed both were beneficial. As it turns out, whole grain is what we should shoot for when making our selections. Multigrain is not necessarily bad for you. It only means that it is made from a variety of grains. To know for sure what it contains, check the ingredients. What you want to see at the front of the ingredient list is "100-percent whole wheat" or "whole grain."

Since we are putting it all together, let's do an exercise using a product that has multigrain on the cover.

1. Go to fooducate.com.

2. Type in the search bar, "Snyder's of Hanover 12 Multi Grain Pretzel Sticks."

3. Check out the letter grade. As of the writing of this book, it has a letter grade of *C-*.

4. Scroll down to Explanations to see why the product received that grade. In a red circle is an exclamation mark. That is your warning. After that icon, it reads, "No grains here." Click the arrow next to, "No grains here." What you will see is helpful information about whole grains. It reads, "Whole grains are a great source of fiber and other nutrients. Fiber is one of the most important nutrients lacking in the modern American diet. Unfortunately, this product does not contain enough whole grains, if any. If there is fiber in here, it's probably added fiber and not naturally occurring. Whole grains are not the only way of consuming fiber, BUT by choosing them instead of processed grains you've made a smart choice. If you'd like to eat a bit better, try for something that contains whole grains."

Eat lean meat and fish. If you are a vegetarian or do not eat fish, do not skip this part. I have you covered too.

- Eat 95–99-percent ground turkey instead of ground beef. Note, the 99-percent ground turkey can be very dry.

A great way to control portions would be to make some turkey meatball muffins.

Choose skinless chicken or turkey breasts. Buy it without the skin or, to save money, remove the skin yourself. Places such as KFC have grilled chicken. If you must eat on the run, get a grilled chicken breast and remove as much of the skin as you can.

- **Eat fish.** Tuna, canned tuna in water, cod, and salmon are great options. Baked or grilled with your Mrs. Dash are the way to go when seasoning. When you are on the go, be prepared with a tuna or salmon packet.

- **Protein for non-meat eaters.** Tofu usually comes to mind, but there are additional options available. Choose from the legume family. That includes peanuts, lentils, beans, and peas. Other good sources for protein for the non-meat eaters are the grain quinoa, nuts and nut butters (such as raw almonds and almond butter), chickpeas, or hemp.

You can easily stash some nuts in a baggie or buy it prepacked to have on the go. Get some unsalted almonds or unsalted walnuts; place them in a bag or container; and have them for a snack. In the next chapter, I will give tips for traveling. Nuts are a great option for such times, especially if flying. Go for the nuts you bring yourself in place of the salted variety given on a plane, if they even provide a free snack.

Keeping-It-Real Solutions and Helpful Tips for Your Struggles, Challenges, and Excuses

I'm not quite sure what the correct portion is. From talking to people, from the reactions I receive on Facebook after posting photos of what I eat on vacation, and from my conversations with my personal trainer, I have come to understand that portion size and portion control are real struggles for some folks. Handling portion size is second nature to me now. As with most of what I know, I did some digging to find a rule of thumb.

Before I get to that, I want to address this notion of a "correct" portion size. I am weary about saying that there is a "correct" size. What you need and what I need are possibly very different. Think of it like this: We have a 250-pound man who wants to get to 200 pounds. To reach his goal weight, he will need to and can consume more food than I could if I still needed to lose fifty pounds. My suggestion to you is not to think of portions as being something right or wrong.

Portions are not limited to how much. Portions also are related to the *what.* Let what you eat be your first line of focus. Use the information that has been shared prior to this chapter to help you with what to eat. As you build upon what to eat, integrate how much. Next is what I did to handle the *how much.*

When I consider how I handled portions while losing weight, I went by the rule of thumb that I found on the Internet: I used the plate and my hand. As I stated above when I suggested eating veggies, I divided the plate in half with an imaginary line. I also have lunch containers to help me do this. I put vegetables on one half of the plate. The remaining half gets split between my protein and starch (carbohydrate other than a vegetable), such as brown rice or a baked sweet potato. One quarter gets protein about the size of my palm. The remaining quarter is for the starch. That is about the size of my fist. Sometimes I would skip the starch altogether. In its place, I would add another vegetable. I typically did that on days that were not dedicated to weight training. For the record, I am speaking in past tense, but I still follow this model today.

Here is something else to note: As you prescribe to what has been shared in this book and start losing weight, you will notice that you will naturally not be able to eat as much. You will get full faster AND from less food. It is truly amazing!! When I started on this subject, I mentioned that handling portion sizes is second nature to me now. When this practice becomes a part of your lifestyle, you will find that you begin setting out your portions naturally too.

But I'm used to only eating twice a day. I'm not that hungry. Oh boy, this one's a doozy. I think I'd die if I only ate twice a day. Of course, I would not die, but I am sure I would be close to passing out. This is not about me though. It is about putting it all together for you so you can get results.

Recall what I have said repeatedly throughout this book, starting from the being: We are all different. Eating five or six small meals a day works for me. As long as eating two meals a day is not your weight-loss method, if all you can manage to eat is two meals a day without being hungry, then eat two meals a day. As I stated above in the last tip, what matters is what you eat and how much of it you eat.

When I was on my journey to losing seventy-five pounds, I had a support system at home: my life partner, Kelly. The woman ate, and still eats, at most, two meals a day. Three meals would be a lot for her. She is rarely ever hungry. She most certainly does not eat just for the sake of eating. In the process of me losing seventy-five pounds, she lost fifteen without trying. She had no goal to lose weight. In fact, neither one of us realized she had, at some point, gained weight. When we look back at pictures now, we can see it, but back then it was not evident.

It was *what* she ate that made the difference. We stopped with the Burger King for dinner. I used to have a Whopper Jr. with fries, and she would have a cheeseburger with fries. When we went to KFC, we traded in fried chicken for grilled chicken. Unlike me, she does not have a love of bread. She did like her gummy bears though. She pretty much eliminated those. We stopped keeping ice cream in the house. If we do have ice cream, it's because she bought it, and it is a very small container and is low-calorie. I am a little more strict than she is, but I also do not like ice cream to that level. We started cooking with olive oil or coconut oil, eating lean meat, and keeping vegetables and fruit in the house. Instead of going out for pizza, we made pizza at home using cauliflower as our "dough." We left the house prepared with snacks, such as carrots, celery, and nuts.

Still, she ate, at most, two meals a day. So, go ahead and keep eating only two meals a day and only when you are hungry. There is nothing wrong with that. The change you more than likely need to make is what you eat for those two meals, as it may be that you are eating too much of the wrong kind of food. If it is not that, you possibly are not eating enough, and your body is reacting to feeling like it does not have enough by letting fat stick around. Take this time to determine which of these is true for you.

It seems like it's too much food. In Chapter 5, I talked about P90X3 laying out a calorie calculation that I believed was too much food. One day, I set aside what I believed and tried the meal plan for the number I had calculated, but I could not stomach all of that food.

There are two ways to know if you are eating too much. The more obvious of the two is that you experience what I experienced: you get full before you finish eating. That is not a bad thing. The other is by measurements: the way your clothes fit, your body measurements, and the scale. Before you make a final judgement, eat what you think is too much for a week. Take your body measurements at the beginning and end of the week. Pay attention to how your clothes fit by the end of the week. Weigh yourself, but do not let that be your determining factor. In "Chapter 11: Move Your Body!" I will go into why in further detail. If your body measurements are bigger and your clothes are fitting tighter, then, as long as you were eating the right kind of food, yes, you ate too much. That is not a bad thing either. The great part about modifying your lifestyle is that you learn what is not working, assess why it is not working, and then make the appropriate adjustments. I did this throughout the process of losing those seventy-five pounds. Those disappointing moments became all the more fulfilling when I figured out what and how to modify.

Just When You had Everything Put Together

Use this chapter as your guide for putting together everything I have shared thus far. Make adjustments where necessary to fit who you are and what your body requires. Do not be afraid to play around and see what works well for you. Most of all, do not get discouraged. This is a process. The greatest part of the process is what you learn along your journey.

You know the "planning and preparation" that keeps coming up? Well, when you are putting it all together and you are starting to make progress, you may face the unexpected. In those times, you need to be prepared for what to do. In the following chapter, I will share tips and tricks to help you through such times. Trust me, over time you will get good at this too. Let's move on to keeping everything in check and, on occasion, putting your foot down.

Don't let anything
or anyone think you
out of what is best
for your well-being.
You do you.

CHAPTER 10

TIPS, TRICKS, AND *OH NO I WON'T*

You are walking with some swag now that you have put everything together, digging into knowing when and why you want to crunch on a greasy, salty bag of chips; you're packing your meals for the week at a scheduled day and time; your grocery basket looks like your health means everything to you, because it does; and you are sharing with family and friends how to be mindful of food labels—then it happens. What is it?

Brace Yourself

You go out to dinner, and they give you a dish big enough to feed a family of four. You show up at the Super Bowl party, and it is a carb fest—and you do not mean the kind from vegetables. These carbs are made with white flour or have been fried. You decide to have a sliver of cake at your sister's birthday celebration, but your aunt is insisting that you look good: "Have a slice of cake." The cake is about three inches wide. This, my friend, is real life. You need to be ready to deal with it while keeping your swag.

101

Ain't No Stoppin' Us Now

When I lost fifty pounds after completing my computer programming courses, I had razor-focus discipline. While eating out with work colleagues or friends, I could easily pass on sharing an order of fries and even bread without a problem. They did not appeal to me.

When I was put in situations where people would otherwise cave, I didn't. At holiday parties and social gatherings or when coworkers set out fat-producing treats, I ignored them without effort. Did I occasionally partake of such indulgences? You bet I did. However, when I did, it was rare. I was able to do that, because living healthy was a lifestyle.

As the beginning of the book stated, I never was on a diet. But how was I able to maintain such focus and discipline when faced with temptation? That is what I address in this chapter. In combination with what I shared in "Chapter 4: Don't Be Caught with Your Pants Down—Be Prepared," about planning and preparation, and "Chapter 9: Putting It All Together," about my eating habits, I implemented these tips and tricks to keep from going down a road that I never want to take again. These are the same tips and tricks that I use today.

So, if you are going to a Super Bowl party, a holiday function—such as Thanksgiving—that is a celebration with food, or any other type of gathering where you believe your defenses are low, give these tips and tricks a try along with what you have learned thus far.

HOW TO DO IT

Share meals. Have you gone out to eat recently? Portion sizes in the U.S. are insanely large. They are too big for one person. No wonder the Organization for Economic Cooperation and Development reported in the fall of 2015, that the United States is home to the most obese population in the Americas, Asia, and Europe.

To no longer be a part of that story, sharing meals is a great technique to help you control your portion sizes when eating out. I also like this method, because, if you cannot decide what to have, you and the person with whom you are eating can share two items, and then—instead of eating everything on your plate—bring home the leftovers. Another bonus is that it helps you save money.

If we know that an establishment is notorious for serving huge portions, we go in with the plan of picking an entrée to share. We even share a salad, as they too can be rather large. When we place the order, we let the wait staff know that we will be sharing. If they do not offer us an additional plate, we request one.

We have not come upon a place that will not allow us to split a meal yet. If that were to happen, we would either order an entrée and an appetizer or small salad, or we would order two entrees, eat half of them, and bring the rest home.

Eat some now, save some for later. Twice above, when speaking of sharing meals, I mentioned taking food home with you. I plucked this idea from that for a reason. I wanted to make sure it stood on its own. Raise your hand or nod your head if in your home growing up you were told to finish ALL the food on your plate. If you did, more than likely you took that rule into adulthood. You no longer have to live by that rule. Whether you are cooking for yourself, out to dinner, or getting something healthy on the go (notice I put the word healthy in there?) go into the meal with the thought of eating some now, but saving some for later. It's all right to not fill your plate or eat everything off the plate.

Drink water to keep you full. "Chapter 8: Water Does a Body and Mind Good," was dedicated to drinking water. Be sure to go back through that chapter. Start the day drinking water. Drink water all day. Drinking water in such a manner will help with the rest of the tips that follow.

Use small plates or containers. Like with sharing meals, using small plates will help you control your portion sizes. The smaller your plate, the less likely you are to pile food on it. Add this tip to what you learned in the previous chapter regarding portion sizes.

I work across the street from a very popular place to eat. Lunch is their busiest time. There is food everywhere. They offer made-to-order salads, sandwiches (really big sandwiches), sushi, and two buffet areas: one for hot food and the other for cold food. I opt for the buffets, because I control how much food I take and the food selection, based on what is available. At each buffet, they provide small and large containers. I always choose the small container. I fill it mostly with vegetables; then I add a protein; and, if they are offering a starch like brown rice, I will put a fistful of that in the container.

Enjoy yourself with small portions. Above, I suggested ways to manage your portions. I am going to take that a step further. Eating to lose or maintain weight, as I have stated before in this book, is not about deprivation. There is nothing wrong with enjoying what you eat, even when it comes to the not-so-healthy stuff. Just keep it to a minimum and limit the frequency.

An occasion when you might enjoy yourself a bit is a holiday such as Thanksgiving. Thanksgiving came through along my journey to losing seventy-five pounds. I had not yet reached that amount, but I had lost a great deal by then. I recall exactly what I had that day: ham, macaroni and cheese, stuffing, corn bread, collard greens, and mixed greens. I also had turkey breast and the grilled salmon that I made and brought with me. The portions of ham, macaroni and cheese, and stuffing were really small. Most of my plate consisted of vegetables. I even had a tiny bit of room for the monkey bread my Aunt Lil made. See, I enjoyed myself, but I did it in small doses. Drinking all that water throughout the day made this quite easy to do.

Start the morning off right. Here are those two words again: planning and preparation. If you have a party or a holiday dinner like Thanksgiving, planning and preparation are a must. Plan to work out the morning of your function. By doing so, you are telling yourself how truly committed you are to your journey, to your process, and to your health and wellness. You are setting yourself up for what you need to do at your gathering. More on that in a little bit. Keep reading.

Bring a healthy dish or two. If you missed it above, I mentioned that I brought grilled salmon to Thanksgiving dinner. Bringing your own meal or dish to a function is a great way to ensure you have a healthy option. This is especially important if you know the last thing that will be at your family's or friend's house is something healthy. Tell me I am not speaking truth.

Eat throughout the day. Whatever the function, make reference to "Chapter 9: Putting It All Together," where I suggest you eat frequent small meals. Start the day with a nice healthy breakfast. Two and a half to three hours later, have a snack or a fruit and a protein, such as yogurt, raw almonds, or cottage cheese. Depending on the time of your function, you may even fit in a light lunch as well. By doing this, you will be hard-pressed to go overboard at dinnertime. The small portions mentioned above will be all you can manage. That is why, though it seemed like I had a lot to eat that Thanksgiving day, I did not. I had planned so sufficiently before arriving that all I could manage to fit in my belly were those small portions. When I say small portions, I mean about the size of the palm of a seven-year-old.

Don't dress the salad. In "Introduction: You Most Certainly Are Not Alone," I mentioned a woman asking me if I lived on salads only. As stated there, I did not live on salads. In fact, I am not a big salad fan. I enjoy hot food, and typically salads do not come with hot toppings.

On the occasion that I do have a salad, I do not smother it with salad dressing. This is because, when left to the place serving it, they are usually a bit too generous with the amount. That can add a lot of unwanted calories, especially if the dressing is a creamy type, such as ranch, blue cheese, or Caesar.

If you are going for a salad, be mindful of what you add to it. Use oil and vinegar or lemon juice as your dressing. If you must have salad dressing, put it in a small cup. I dip my fork in it and let a little coat the prongs, and then I pick up a forkful of mixed greens, spinach, or kale. Prong dipping limits the amount of dressing you use. In turn, that helps control the added calories from fatty dressings. When dining out, be sure to ask for it on the side and use the fork trick.

Eating-out modifications. In "Chapter 4: Don't Be Caught with Your Pants Down—Be Prepared," I mentioned asking that dishes be modified when eating out. Asking for the salad dressing on the side is not the only modification I make when going out to eat. Keep these tips at the forefront of your mind. In fact, go into the dining experience prepared to make these types of modifications.

If grilled chicken comes topped with sauce or butter, ask for the chicken without the sauce. If a dish comes with fries of any kind, including sweet potato fries (hello, they are fried!), ask to substitute them with a small mixed-green salad (I have learned the hard way that places will give you a salad made with iceberg and call that baby a mixed salad—grr!!) or with a vegetable.

If the dish comes with white rice or mashed potatoes, look for their list of sides or the sides that come with other dishes. My experience is that, if a place is offering white rice, a vegetable is probably your only other option. You could always lean out for hope of quinoa or brown rice, but do not hold your breath. Instead, go for another vegetable or a baked potato (no butter, no sour cream, and no salt) in place of the white rice. "Chapter 3: Get That C.R.A.P. Out of My House," touches on the types of carbohydrates you should be seeking. Baked potatoes offer some pretty awesome nutritional benefits; however, once mashed, many places are probably going to whip those potatoes up with a lot of butter. Since you do not know for sure what they do, follow the same suggestions that I provided for the white rice.

No cheating required. Cheating sounds so naughty. It sounds as if you have something to hide. Treats every now and then are fine. They only become problematic when you are consuming them more times than not. Enjoy a treat in moderation rather than every day, several times a day. Have nibbles, not huge helpings.

On this subject of treats, Shaun T, the fitness trainer and motivator who encourages us to dig deeper and trust and believe, says he lives by what he calls the 85/15 rule. Eighty-five percent of the food he eats is healthy. He calls the remaining fifteen percent "fun foods." Shaun suggests we take the following steps:

1. Draw a line down the center of a sheet of paper.

2. On the left side, label it Healthy Foods.

3. List the healthy foods that you like.

4. On the right side, label it Fun Foods.

5. List some of the fun foods you love.

6. Eat more foods from the healthy food list than from the fun food list.[6]

If you are stretched for determining healthy foods to add to your list, I provide you with a list of healthy foods at pamelaburke.com/dietfreeme-resources.

If you fear you cannot eat treats in moderation or by Shaun's method, keep temptation foods out of your house. We covered that in Chapter 3. Here is why: If you keep your aunt's to-die-for sweet potato pie out of your house, you will avoid sneaking more than a slice of that pie because you could not say *no*. Speaking of which, check out the next tip.

---

[6] Shaun T. "Treat Not Cheat." *Healthyway*. Healthyway, 2016. Web. 20 May 2016. http://www.healthyway.com/content/treat-not-cheat.

Smile, and then say, "Thank You, I'm good." Then repeat. It is quite possible that you have a family much like mine; they love to eat. What I know about mine—and this may be true of yours—is that there is going to be a family member who will believe I have not eaten enough. If so, they are going to pester you and pester you about eating more.

Aunt Ella is going to say, "Girl, you barely ate. Go get yourself some more." And she is going to keep saying it. Uncle Earl is going to tell you, "Baby, you ain't got no meat on them bones. Go get some more of your Aunt Doris' yams and macaroni and cheese." (Meanwhile, you know you have another thirty-plus pounds to lose.) Do you know what you are going to do, because you had a plan coming into the day? You are going to keep being polite and let them know that you are done. If you feel you cannot take it, kindly excuse yourself from the table.

Always have healthy snack options available. A question was once posed by a work colleague on our company forum: "How do you fight snacking when coworkers bring cookies, cakes, sandwiches, soda, etc.?" While throwing evil glares, using voodoo dolls, and "accidentally" spilling water on the treats of said colleagues are options, that is not, of course, what you should do. More civilized suggestions were offered on the forum. Those responses were very much in line with my own. In fact, I have shared many already. Drink water (Chapter 8). Always have healthy snack options available. That is in line with what I said above about bringing your own healthy options to a party. Lastly, as noted above, an occasional treat is not a bad thing. You are better off having a small treat than gorging on several.

Rev up the workouts. If you are not currently working out, start. If you are already working out, up the intensity. On those special-occasion days when you might eat atypically, add in a second workout one day. That is the strategy I used the Thanksgiving I mentioned earlier: I went for an eight-mile run in the morning, and, before getting ready for dinner, I did a Shaun T workout.

Let your body know you love it. CAUTION: Do not do too much too fast. I will talk more about working out in the next chapter.

If Only Changing Your Diet Were Enough

This book has been heavily focused on managing a healthy lifestyle centered around your diet. That was intentional. The focus is on what people let me know gave them the most fits: handling eating. Even so, I cannot end this book without speaking about the other component of my weight-loss success: exercise. I have already mentioned exercise a little, but the next chapter will give more specifics in relation to what I did. Get ready to move your body!

Doing something
is always better
than nothing.
Strive to do something.

CHAPTER 11

MOVE YOUR BODY!

We are nearing the finish line of this book. By now, you know what I am going to say, right? Your planning and preparation are so on point now; you are so prepared that you set time to plan and prepare. I do not mean to come off like a broken record. I aim to help you help yourself. You just completed setting tactics to keep from squashing your progress. Now we will add a little more to that success. I encourage you to move your body.

Born to Run and Play

Growing up, I was a skinny kid. I did not eat very much, because I did not like very much. I rarely ever tried anything new. What I did do as a kid, though, was spend my time outside playing. Always the competitive person, I raced the boys in the neighborhood by foot and on my bike. I would climb fences and trees, even though every time I got up, I was terrified of coming back down because of my fear of falling and fear of heights.

As I got older, I took part in team sports. I played soccer, basketball, and softball, and, when I gave up softball, because I found it boring, I joined the track team. Exercise during that time was natural. It came with the territory.

Even in college, I kept in shape. During my sophomore year of college, I was a walk-on with the basketball team. On occasion, I also played recreation basketball. I remained rather thin up through my late twenties.

No Time for Playtime

By my early twenties, soon after graduating from college, my life shifted. Most of my day was spent sitting behind a desk. My physical activity had decreased, but it had no effect on my weight. Heck, even eating fries, burgers, and pizza had no effect on me. Once I hit thirty, the combination of that sort of diet and lack of exercise caught up to me. Slowly, I was inching out of my size eight into bigger sizes.

Things did not get out of hand until I was knee-deep into my computer programming studies. As I shared earlier, there was barely any sleep for me, and there was, for certain, very little exercise. The walk from the train to the office was not giving me the calorie burn needed to help combat my unhealthy, sedentary lifestyle. The same story would hold true when I went through my master's degree program in my early forties. Both left me significantly overweight.

Make Time for Workout Time

Changing my eating habits made a significant difference, but that alone is not what attributed to my healthier lifestyle. Adding exercise back into my life also attributed to it. Exercise is the focus in this chapter.

HOW TO DO IT

Move your body with high-intensity workouts. Yes, changing your eating habits to a healthier lifestyle will help you lose weight. Just eliminate sugar from your diet and you will see that. Moving your body with exercise will help the weight loss along a tad bit faster. That is especially the case when you work out using high-intensity exercises. (Be sure to consult your physician before starting any new workout program.)

High-intensity exercises keep the heart rate up. This will help you burn more calories. When we burn more calories than we take into our bodies, we lose weight. We have covered that a couple of times now. With high-intensity workouts, you do not need to do hours of exercise to get results.

If your form of exercise is walking a comfortable stroll, unless you are morbidly obese, that is not high-intensity, and you will have to walk for several hours to see results. If that is what your doctor prescribes for you, then be sure to follow doctor's orders.

Also know, especially if you are just starting with a workout program, high-intensity is not created equal. What looks like high-intensity for one person may not be intense for another person, or it may be too intense for yet another person. Do the best that you can. Remain consistent. (More on that in a moment.) In time, your level of intensity will increase. Another thing to note is that, with high-intensity workouts, you can work out in as little as twenty-five to thirty minutes, consistently, and see results. Gone are the days of hour-plus long workouts.

Be consistent. The best way to see results from your workouts is by being consistent with them. Consistency is working out a minimum of three times every week. If you are doing the right kind of exercises, anything over thirty minutes for each day that you exercise is not necessary. I, for example, worked out five or six times a week while losing weight. After losing the weight, the second go-around, I scaled back to three or four times per week. While writing this book, I went back to five or six times per week.

Consistency makes a huge difference in your results as well as your progress. Before losing weight, I could not do most of the INSANITY workouts by Shaun T. I could barely do two push-ups because I was so weak, and I could not do a decent looking burpee. Consistency changed that.

113

I can now get through an INSANITY workout without as much of a problem, though they are still challenging. I push myself to be better than the last time. I now do incline push-ups and advanced forms of burpees. For the advanced version, my personal trainer has me squat with twenty-pound weights, go down into a push-up, do alternate rows while in the plank position, and then pop back up from a squat position into a shoulder press and repeat it all again for thirty to forty-five seconds.

Without consistency, I would not have been able to progress to that level. Not only did I lose weight, but I also gained strength and confidence. When you remain consistent, you can enjoy the same transformative experience.

Put yourself first: Make working out routine. Above, I talked about working out consistently. Below, I will talk about planning your workout schedule. Before moving on, take this time to set in your mind that, from this moment forward, you will put yourself first. You will make working out, healthy eating, and mental strength your priorities.

I have watched family members, friends, and acquaintances put work, spouses, children, and parents before their own well-being. I have done the same. We are no benefit to the ones we love or for our employers (if we work for someone else) when we do not make our health and wellness priorities.

Now that my health and wellness are priorities, working out is a routine part of my life. If I skip a workout, or if I consider skipping one, it feels much like forgetting to brush my teeth. I cannot recall a time when I have done that. Do you get my point? Working out is that important to me.

I limit my TV time to get in a workout. I schedule morning meetings at times that will allow me to work out first. When someone schedules a meeting at a time that interferes with my ability to work out, I check to see if it can be held at a later time. If that is not possible, I make adjustments. (See below for more on making adjustments.) I do this because, when I work out, I get clarity for my work, for my writing, and for what I want to accomplish in life. Running, for example, releases creativity in me.

Even if my schedule only allows me to get in a five-, ten-, or twelve-minute workout, I will squeeze it in. Again, working out is that important to me. My mentality is that doing something is better than doing nothing. Ingrain that type of thinking too, and you will be a benefit to those around you.

Schedule time to work out. Oh, the dreaded workout schedule. There is no one-size-fits-all here. Adjust your schedule accordingly until you strike something that allows you to remain consistent. I work out before work. I discovered that exercising in the morning, before work, gave me the best guarantee that I would work out. It also helps that I am a morning person.

Working out during lunch was an option, especially since our office has a gym with showers, but once I took off my work clothes, I did not want to put them back on again. All I wanted to do was shower and head home.

Waiting until after work to exercise would not allow me to remain consistent. My job is not 9:00–5:00. It is 9:00 until whenever I leave. It is really difficult to have a consistent workout schedule when such is the case.

Another issue that I had was being too tired to work out after work. Even if I managed to drag myself to a workout, I did not get as much out of it. I was too mentally and physically fatigued to perform at my best.

Morning workouts may not be your thing. For example, my sister is quite the opposite of me. She can start a workout—yoga being her exercise regime of choice—at 10:00 at night. At that hour, I am already sleeping. She is at her best in the late evening. Me—not so much.

In addition to the time of day, also determine which days of the week work best for you. Monday mornings are tough for me, but I have yet to discover why. In order to get in six days, I push through the Monday-morning workout, or I give up on it and work out on Sunday before heading to church. On Wednesday and Friday, I work out with my personal trainer. Then on Tuesday, Thursday, and Saturday, I am on my own. Typically, I do some form of cardio on those days. I will discuss my preferred forms of workouts next.

The key for you is to look at your calendar, understand what days of the week are optimal, and then schedule what workouts you will do on what days and for how long.

Be willing to adjust. There are times when my schedule will not allow me to work out at my planned time. Such times are when a work meeting is scheduled too early in the day for me to work out at my usual time. There are also occurrences when I am leaving for an early flight to go on vacation—sometimes waking up as early as 2:30 or 3:00 in the morning to start getting ready to head to the airport. There is no time to work out. And even I, living by the creed that doing something is better than doing nothing, am too dang sleepy to begin thinking about putting in even a minute of exercise at that hour. Whatever the reason may be, I make adjustments.

During the journey to losing seventy-five pounds, there would be a day in the week where I worked out twice on that day. Then—and now—if Sunday was my off day, I would work out on a Sunday to make up for a missed day. On rare occasions, I would work out after work, if my schedule allowed it. If all else failed, I would skip the workout and focus on ramping things up the following week. If I could only get in three workouts one week, it was what it was. I was not aiming for perfection. I was aiming for doing the best that I could to make working out consistently a part of my life. If life dictates that you make adjustments, then make adjustments. You can still be consistent and adjust.

Choose a workout regime that challenges you but that you like. Making time to work out, on its own, can be a challenge. There is no need to add to it by forcing yourself to do exercises that you loathe. That is not to say that you avoid a particular exercise because you do not like it. It means there is a difference between hating burpees and hating to run on a treadmill. I hated burpees because they were a challenge. That was no reason to not do them. In fact, burpees are a great full-body, high-intensity exercise. Like with most things, the more I did them, the better I got at them. At this point, a regular burpee is not all that challenging anymore. Now, as for the treadmill, I hate running on them—HATE. IT. But, I do like running. As a matter of fact, hands down, running outside is my workout method of choice. If you don't like running, inside or out, by all means, do not use running as your mode of exercise.

If you try to use an exercise that you do not like as a way to help you lose weight, it won't be long until you stop doing that exercise. Worse yet, you may never reach your weight-loss goal. Play with workout routines and exercises until you determine what works for you. In the trying, you are still getting a workout. There are plenty of ways to get your body moving, so determine the exercises that are for you.

The same idea holds true about whether or not you get a gym membership to exercise. Overall, I hate the whole gym experience. That is why I don't have a membership. If I am not running, I am strength training or doing high-intensity interval training (HIIT) workouts with my personal trainer, or I am working out to a DVD. Shaun T is my man. His INSANITY workouts are challenging and long. I never made it to his second level of INSANITY workouts, because they are too long. Too long, to me, is anything over thirty minutes. That is what I mean when I say learn what works for you. Shaun T and Beachbody, for whom he works, figured out that most people are like me. We ain't got time for that (workouts over thirty minutes). That is why Shaun T now has T25 and INSANITY Max:30. I like those workouts, because I am challenged in short spurts.

What is great too about Shaun T is that he includes a modifier in his workout routines. If you cannot yet go full-out, Shaun T has you covered with the modifier. The movements have been modified, but, for your fitness level, the exercises are more than likely still intense. Shaun T may not fit you.

There are plenty of at-home DVDs. Search YouTube or do a Google search to see the type of instruction that works best for your temperament. I like to be pushed and not have someone smiling and giggling when I work out. But that may be exactly what you need. Again, it takes time and experience to learn which workouts work best for you. Enjoy the journey while you learn.

Embrace your muscles by working your muscles. A great way to lose weight, in addition to eating healthy, is by incorporating strength/weight training into your workout routine. In this section, I will be using strength training and weight training interchangeably.

If you think muscle weighs more than fat, fear muscle bulk, or are solely focused on the number on the scale, let those thoughts go. You want to include weight training as a part of your weight-loss and weight-maintenance regime because of the benefits of strength training.

Here is why: A pound of muscle burns more fat than a pound of fat. Long after you finish working out, muscle is still working to burn calories. If you only do cardio, you are losing muscle, thus depleting your calorie-burning machine that helps you lose weight. Muscle is also more dense than fat. Thus, a pound of muscle takes up less physical space than does a pound of fat. As your body measurements decrease, so does your body-fat percentage. What's cool about that is the physical space that your body takes up also decreases. That change in your body composition means you can weigh more and still fit into a smaller size. How cool is that?! So, back in "Chapter 9: Putting It All Together," if you are concerned that you may be eating too much, this was the section I was referring to when talking about body measurements.

That is what I experienced after losing the seventy-five pounds. My goal was to get into a size eight. In order to do that, I aimed to lose eighty-five pounds. I was able to get into my size eights again while holding on to ten additional pounds. That was all because of the change in my body composition, aided by strength training. This is why I highly recommend that you not rely solely on cardio. Include strength training to your exercise too.

Don't take a workout vacation on vacation. When you go on vacation, you may be tempted to take a vacation from everything. That includes a vacation

118

from working out. Don't do it! Keep working out as part of your routine. You do not want to run the risk of not restarting when you return from vacation.

While you are away from home, include excursions that require activities such as walking, hiking, swimming, playing sports, or rowing. On a cruise vacation to Alaska, that is what I did. Every morning, I got up at the same time as I would at home. On weight-training days, I used the gym on the ship. On running days, I ran on the track on the ship. When we docked, I booked an ice trekking excursion (that was a beautiful experience—even in the cold, I was sweating) at one location and a kayaking excursion at another.

If you will be staying in a hotel while away, even if it is not a vacation, pick a hotel with gym equipment and work out there. If you like running, drive around to plan a route to run or scope out a local park. I have done all of these when I am away from home. If I am staying at a place that does not have a gym, I bring my gym with me. That gym is a bag with resistance bands. That is what it looks like when you make your health a priority.

Listen to your body: rest. Up to this point, the focus has been on moving your body. To obtain weight-loss results and to maintain your weight, eating right and exercising are a one-two punch. What makes them more effective is to be certain to get your rest. When you are exercising consistently, your body needs time to recover. Your muscles need time to repair themselves after you have broken them down with weight training. We covered that in the last tip. Sleep is the best way to get that rest. How much sleep we need varies by person. Experience tells me I need seven to eight hours of sleep. Anything less than that and I am sluggish; I struggle to get up for workouts, causing me to limit my workout time sometimes; or my workout is compromised. The workout looks ugly, or I struggle through exercises that normally would not give me a problem.

There are times, though, when you are eating well, working out consistently, and getting the proper amount of rest (for you), but you still feel out of sorts. You feel like you have slowed down. You may struggle to think clearly. You feel tired. That is your body talking to you. Your body is letting you know you need rest. I have done that by taking off a day or two from workouts. I have also taken a week where I lessen the intensity of my workouts by doing light yoga and taking walks. I never take off for too long. I get my rest, and then I get back to the routine.

Keeping-It-Real Solutions and Helpful Tips for Your Struggles, Challenges, and Excuses

I do not have time to work out. I too did not have time to work out, until I made time to work out. We all have twenty-four hours in our day. How do you make more time than that? You don't, because we can't. What you can do, however, is assess where you spend your time and on what.

Above, I mentioned that I work out in the morning before work. I also shared why other times of day, during lunch and after work, do not work for me. Determining that in the morning before work was the best time for me to work out was a process.

I had to, first, honestly assess how I was spending my time. Before working out became my lifestyle, my mornings were spent sleeping in the bed, checking emails, searching my Facebook feed, and finding any other distraction other than working out. My next course of action was to try exercising different times of the day. During a work week, as I have mentioned, after work was out. I never knew when I was leaving work. I found myself either too tired or canceling my workout plans to finish up something at the office. Here is what I recommend to help you determine your optimal workout time.

1. **Take an assessment.** Assess where you spend your time and on what. For a week, chart your activity.
2. **Track your time.** Note how much time you spend on those activities.

3. **Categorize where you spend your time.** For each activity, tag it with *absolutely necessary, could have delegated, could have waited*, or *made me feel better.*

- *Absolutely necessary* could be time you spent driving yourself to work, working, or attending a priority function, such as a mandatory meeting or a child's practice or game.

- *Could have delegated* is pretty obvious. It is something you could have given someone else to do.

- *Could have waited* is something that did not need to be done at that moment. For example, if you have a goal to read a book, that could be done at a different, specified, planned time. I sometimes use my bus rides home from work for reading.

- *Made me feel better* are those activities that we do to avoid something we should be doing, like exercising (hint hint). Such activities are spending time on social media, watching television, or talking on the phone or texting. Another way to think of *made me feel better* is idle time. It is that time you spend on an activity that has no significance.

4. **Reassess the *absolutely necessary* time.** Was it really absolutely necessary? If yes, fine. If not, move it to the appropriate category.

5. **Review and repeat.** Review all times other than *absolutely necessary.*

6. **Review the time spent in each category.** How much time did you spend in those areas? Note that time; then note what time of the day, and on what days, you have the most time or some available pockets of time.

7. **Set your day and time to work out.** Use that time to determine the best days and times to exercise.

Know this: Any amount of time you put forth to make time for working out and to take care of your well-being is better than making no time at all.

That is well and good, but I still do not have time to work out. Yes, you do have time. You may be challenged, but, by being flexible with your time and creativity, you can make time for workouts where you can fit them in. I wrote a blog post—at canwilldone.com—with the headline, "How do you find time to work out? – 5 Ways to Get It In." The post begins with:

Are you saying, "Forget about how I find time to work out, what about what if there is no time in my day to work out?"

Is that your life? Are you so insanely busy that you have determined there is no possible way that you have time to exercise – not in the morning, not in the noon day, not in the evening, no time of day?

I use a work colleague as an example of someone who is challenged to find time to work out. She could not work out in the morning before work, since she had to get up at 4:00 a.m. just to make it to the train. After work, workouts were out too. As a project manager, she typically works late. With work meetings throughout the day, even going to the gym at work is not an option. I put myself in her shoes to determine what I would do if I were her. My solution was to get it in where I could fit it in. Here is a handful of my suggestions.

1. **Be flexible.** I said it above: Doing something is far better than doing nothing. Rather than thinking with a mindset of all-or-nothing ("If I cannot do a thirty-minute workout, then I cannot do anything."), tell yourself you will make the most of the time you have available throughout the day.

2. **Be creative, always thinking of ways to move your body.** In line with being flexible, ramp up your creative juices. Think to yourself:

   • "I have five to ten minutes available in the morning; I will do five to ten minutes of T25."

- "Instead of parking close to the building, I will park as far away as possible and briskly walk to the building."

- "I have a half-hour between meetings in the morning; I will take a brisk walk around the building while I check emails on my phone."

- "My daughter has a baseball game after work. Rather than sitting around watching, I will take a run around the bases of an open field or take a run around the play area. I will ask my friend to join me, since she has said she needs to lose weight too."

3. **Walk everywhere.** Give yourself a reason to walk. Instead of sitting at your desk for hours at a time, set a timer to get up at thirty-minute intervals to go for a short, brisk walk. Use some of the walking examples used above. Take the stairs rather than the elevator. Again, be creative.

4. **Use housework to your advantage.** Work around the house is a form of exercise. Did you ever take note of that? Clean the bathroom; sweep, mop, or vacuum the floors; rake leaves; push a handheld lawnmower; paint rooms; wash dishes by hand; or cook for yourself. All of these keep your body moving, thus adding more calorie burning to your day.

5. **Create a challenge.** I referenced in "Chapter 5: Tools of the Trade—the Go-To Technology," that I use a tracking device called Misfit. It tracks my steps and number of calories burned. There are all types of devices that do the same—Fitbit, Garmin vivofit, and Nike+ are just some of the devices currently available. You can use such a device to give yourself a daily, weekly, and monthly challenge.

You may have heard about setting a goal to walk 10,000 steps. That is a great goal for someone starting out. That can be your initial goal. If you already have achieved 10,000 steps on a regular basis, challenge yourself to do more. Up the count by 2,000 additional steps. Or aim to burn more calories from week to week.

Because of my level of fitness and the types of activities I did, I had days where I would surpass 25,000 steps. The Misfit has a point system. Rather than try to reach a certain number of steps, I set a goal to reach a certain number of points a day. Depending on the type of workout I had planned for the day, I would adjust the points goal—meaning, on running days, I would increase the points. That was because a five-mile run could easily get me to my points goal for a weight-training day. Have fun with the process.

The more you make these types of adjustments in your life, the better you will get at making them.

Reward yourself with doing more of what helped you achieve your goal.

CHAPTER 12

AND, IN CONCLUSION, MAKE SURE YOU STAY ON TOP

As the chorus from the R&B group Boyz II Men says, "We've come to the end of the road." With this entry, the chapters of *Diet-Free Me* have come to a close. Even so, the book and its contents are here whenever you need them. It is my belief, from my own experience and from observation, that we focus so much on losing weight that we forget to give focus, or we do not realize we need to give focus, to what we should do after we lose the weight. My advice to you is, for whatever stage you are on along your journey to weight loss and better overall health for a lifetime, be prepared.

In life, we may want everything now, but this journey is a process. In the introduction, I told you what I realized: To even begin living your weight-loss journey, it requires a change in how you think. The process begins in your mind. Therefore, change your way of thinking. Take one step at a time, starting with digging deeper ("Chapter 2: When You Have Had Enough, Dig Deep into Your *Why?*") by working on self-introspection.

PAMELA BURKE

Leave no doubt that you will have healthy options around, with a home full of wholesome, good-for-your-health food selections ("Chapter 3: Get That C.R.A.P. Out of My House").

By preparing and planning your own meals, you can be certain you won't be caught with your pants down ("Chapter 4: Don't Be Caught with Your Pants Down—Be Prepared).

Stay close to your tools of the trade ("Chapter 5: Tools of the Trade— the Go-To Technology"). MyFitnessPal and Fooducate will act as your personal assistants.

With those tools, planning and preparation, you know you will be a grocery-shopping master by going on every trip to the store with your foolproof strategy ("Chapter 6: From Grocery-Shopping Flunky to Master Shopper").

No matter if it is while grocery shopping, in line to buy a new gadget or paper supplies, or on a trip to a convenience store, get a good laugh and proudly walk out of the store knowing you were not fooled by label trickery ("Chapter 7: Don't Be Fooled").

Drink so much water you feel like you are going to bust, but don't mind it, since you know you are doing your body and mind good with every ounce ("Chapter 8: Water Does a Body and Mind Good").

Put digging deeper, planning and preparation, your tools, savvy shopping, and water consumption all together to make eating the right foods a no-brainer ("Chapter 9: Putting It All Together").

Going to a party or out to eat, or have coworkers who insist on bringing fattening treats to work? No worries. You are armed with tips and tricks to make it easy for you to resist ("Chapter 10: Tips, Tricks, and *Oh No I Won't*").

You'll really put it all together and see amazing results, since, along with planning and preparing what you eat, you'll also be planning and preparing to keep your body moving through consistent exercise ("Chapter 11: Move Your Body!").

128

As I stated in the opening of the book, our lives and bodies are unique; therefore, there is no one-size-fits-all. For any—or all—of the above, make adjustments where you need them to fit your life and your body.

I close with this: Mia Hamm, former American soccer player, two-time Women's World Cup winner, and two-time Olympic gold medalist said, "It is more difficult to stay on top than to get there." Yes, sometimes along this journey, you may feel as though it is hard and maintaining your new weight may seem even harder, but you know what? Making your mental and physical health a priority is well worth the challenge. Besides, the confidence and strength you gain from your challenges will trump "easy" every time. That struggle you were saying was real—you now have the power and the confidence to put an end to such struggles, diet-free, with no pills, body wraps, saunas, plastic suits, or fad diets. You're now ready and well-prepared to stay on top by choosing to embrace a healthy lifestyle for a lifetime. In the process, you will likely lose weight. That's the bonus. The person you become is the real prize. Before you know it, people will be asking you, "How'd you do it?"

BIBLIOGRAPHY

"12 Deadly Workout Sins." *Body for Life*. Abbott Laboratories, 2014. Web. 28 May 2016. http://bodyforlife.com/library/articles/training/12-deadly-workout-sins.

"Ask the Dietitian: What's the Best Carb, Protein and Fat Breakdown for Weight Loss?" *hellohealthy*. MyFitnessPal, Inc., 3 February 2015. Web. 18 April 2016. http://blog.myfitnesspal.com/ask-the-dietitian-whats-the-best-carb-protein-and-fat-breakdown-for-weight-loss/.

"Baked Lays." *Mr. Johnson's Blog*. N.p., February 2012. Web. 24 January 2016. https://nosajnawk.files.wordpress.com/2012/02/bakedlays.jpg.

"Balancing Carbs, Protein, and Fat." *GroupHealth*. Group Health Cooperative, n.d. Web. 23 May 2016. http://www.ghc.org/healthAndWellness/?item=/common/healthAndWellness/conditions/diabetes/foodBalancing.html.

Barnes, Zahra. "Q&A: What's the Difference Between Multigrain, Whole Grain, and Whole Wheat?" *Women's Health*. Rodale Inc., 22 August 2014. Web. 30 January 2016. http://www.womenshealthmag.com/food/whole-wheat-vs-whole-grain-vs-multigrain.

Benfit, Emily. "Why I Hate the '5-Ingredient Rule.'" *Butter Believer*. Butter Believer, 19 April 2013. Web. 8 February 2016. http://butterbeliever.com/why-i-hate-the-5-ingredient-rule/.

Bob's Red Mill. Bob's Red Mill Natural Foods. Web. 1 May 2016. http://www.bobsredmill.com/organic-thick-rolled-oats.html.

Brody, Jane E. "Why Your Workout Should Be High-Intensity." *The New York Times.* The New York Times Company, 26 January 2015. Web. 26 May 2016. http://well.blogs.nytimes.com/2015/01/26/sweaty-answer-to-chronic-illness/?_r=0.

"Carbohydrates: Simple versus Complex." *NutritionMD.* NutritionMD, n.d. Web. 3 April 2016. http://www.nutritionmd.org/nutrition_tips/nutrition_tips_understand_foods/carbs_versus.html.

Cherney, Kristeen. "Simple Carbohydrates vs. Complex Carbohydrates." *Healthline.* Healthline Media, n.d. Web. 4 May 2016. http://www.healthline.com/health/food-nutrition/simple-carbohydrates-complex-carbohydrates.

"The Difference Between Whole Grains & Whole Wheat [Bread Miniseries Part 2/4]." *Fooducate.* Fooducate LTD, 10 March 2015. Web. 30 January 2016. http://blog.fooducate.com/2015/03/10/the-difference-between-whole-grains-whole-wheat-bread-miniseries-part-24/.

"Fad Diets." *UPMC.* UPMC. Web. 27 March 2016. http://www.upmc.com/patients-visitors/education/nutrition/pages/fad-diets.aspx.

"Fiening." *Urban Dictionary.* Urban Dictionary. Web. 23 May 2016. http://www.urbandictionary.com/define.php?term=Fiening.

Fooducate. Fooducate LTD. Web. 1 May 2016. http://www.fooducate.com/.

Gunnars, Kris. "6 Reasons Why Gluten is Bad For Some People." *Authority Nutrition.* Authority Nutrition, November 2013. Web. 23 May 2016.

https://authoritynutrition.com/6-shocking-reasons-why-gluten-is-bad/.

Gunnars, Kris. "The 20 Most Weight Loss Friendly Foods on The Planet." *Authority Nutrition.* Authority Nutrition, 2014. Web. 2 December 2015. https://authoritynutrition.com/20-most-weight-loss-friendly-foods/.

Gunnars, Kris. "Why Ezekiel Bread is The Healthiest Bread You Can Eat." *Authority Nutrition.* Authority Nutrition, April 2016. Web. 3 April 2016. https://authoritynutrition.com/ezekiel-bread/.

"Health." *Merriam-Webster.* Merriam-Webster, Incorporated. Web. 27 March 2016. http://www.merriam-webster.com/dictionary/health.

"Healthy." *Merriam-Webster.* Merriam-Webster, Incorporated. Web. 27 March 2016. http://www.merriam-webster.com/dictionary/healthy.

"High Fructose Corn Syrup: Questions and Answers." *FDA.* U.S. Food and Drug Administration, n.d. Web. 26 May 2016. http://www.fda.gov/Food/IngredientsPackagingLabeling/FoodAdditiv esIngredients/ucm324856.htm.

"How to Replace Refined Carbohydrates." *SFGate.* N.p., n.d. Web. 7 November 2015. http://healthyeating.sfgate.com/replace-refined-carbohydrates-6215.html.

"If Big Name Companies Were More 'Honest' With Their Branding." *B&T.* The Misfits Media Company Pty Limited, 21 April 2016. Web. 30 April 2016. http://www.bandt.com.au/marketing/big-name-companies-honest-branding.

Kravitz, Len. "High-Intensity Interval Training." *ACSM.* American College of Sports Medicine, 2014. Web. 26 May 2016. https://www.acsm.org/docs/brochures/high-intensity-interval-training.pdf.

"Lifestyle." *Merriam-Webster.* Merriam-Webster, Incorporated. Web. 27 March 2016. http://www.merriam-webster.com/dictionary/lifestyle.

"Macronutrients: the Importance of Carbohydrate, Protein, and Fat." *McKinley Health Center—University of Illinois.* The Board of Trustees of the University of Illinois, 2014. Web. 26 May 2016. http://www.mckinley.illinois.edu/handouts/macronutrients.htm.

Magee, Elaine. "3 Meals a Day or 6 Smaller Meals? Experts Weigh the Pros and Cons." *MedicineNet.* MedicineNet, Inc, n.d. Web. 23 May 2016. http://www.medicinenet.com/script/main/art.asp?articlekey=56254.

McMillen, Matt. "Paleo Diet (Caveman Diet) Review, Foods List, and More." *WebMD.* WebMD, LLC. Web. 23 May 2016. http://www.webmd.com/diet/a-z/paleo-diet.

MyFitnessPal. MyFitnessPal, Inc. Web. 18 April 2016. https://www.myfitnesspal.com/.

"Nutritional Information." *TGI Friday's.* TGI Friday's Inc, n.d. Web. 16 April 2016. https://www.tgifridays.com/nutrition.pdf.

Penner, Elle. "Is Cornstarch Bad For Me?" *According to Elle.* According to Elle, 21 September 2012. Web. 23 May 2016. http://www.accordingtoelle.com/cornstarch-what-is-it-and-is-it-bad-for-me/.

Phillips, Bill, and Michael D'Orso. *Body for Life: 12 Weeks to Mental and Physical Strength.* New York: HarperCollins Publishers, 1999. Print.

"Q&A: 'Toxic' effects of sugar: should we be afraid of fructose?" *BioMed Central.* BioMed Central Ltd, 21 May 2012. Web. 14 March 2016. http://bmcbiol.biomedcentral.com/articles/10.1186/1741-7007-10-42.

Quinn, Elizabeth. "Why Athletes Need Rest and Recovery After Exercise." *Verywell.* About, Inc, 7 April 2016. Web. 28 May 2016. https://www.verywell.com/the-benefits-of-rest-and-recovery-after-exercise-3120575.

"Real Food Defined." *Eat Good 4 Life.* Eat Good 4 Life, n.d. Web. 8 February 2016. http://www.eatgood4life.com/real-food-defined/.

Sanders, Jeff. *The 5 AM Miracle: Dominate Your Day before Breakfast.* Berkeley, CA: Ulysses Press, 2015. Print.

Schwartz, Jay. "Do You Burn More Calories When Your Heart Beats Faster?" *AZ Central.* N.p., n.d. Web. 27 May 2016. http://healthyliving.azcentral.com/burn-calories-heart-beats-faster-8069.html.

Shaun T. "Treat Not Cheat." *Healthyway.* Healthyway, 2016. Web. 20 May 2016. http://www.healthyway.com/content/treat-not-cheat.

"Slide Show: Low-calorie-density Foods for Weight Control." *Mayo Clinic.* Mayo Foundation for Medical Education and Research, n.d. Web. 10 January 2016. http://www.mayoclinic.org/healthy-lifestyle/weight-loss/multimedia/low-calorie-foods/sls-20076175.

"SlimFast™ | How It Works." *SlimFast.* SlimFast. Web. 15 May 2016. http://slimfast.ca/how-it-works.

"Snyder's of Hanover Pretzel Sticks, 8 Grains & Seeds." *Fooducate.* Fooducate LTD. Web. 1 May 2016. http://www.fooducate.com/app#!page=product&id=76A53EDA-E112-11DF-A102-FEFD45A4D471.

Spano, Marie. "What Does 'Eating Clean' Really Mean?" *Bodybuilding.com.* Bodybuilding.com, LLC, 2015. Web. 16 March 2016. http://www.bodybuilding.com/fun/what-does-eating-clean-really-mean.

Stewart, Kristen. "Does Muscle Weigh More Than Fat?" *Everyday Health.*
Everyday Health Media, n.d. Web. 22 July 2015.
http://www.everydayhealth.com/weight/busting-the-muscle-weighs-
more-than-fat-myth.aspx.

"Strawberry Twizzlers Twists." *Hershey.* The Hershey Company. Web. 24
January 2016. https://www.thehersheycompany.com/brands/twizzlers-
twists/strawberry.aspx.

Taub-Dix, Bonnie. "5 Reasons You Should Eat Oatmeal Every Day."
Everyday Health. Everyday Health Media, LLC, 28 October 2014.
Web. 1 May 2016. http://www.everydayhealth.com/columns/bonnie-
taub-dix-nutrition-intuition/reasons-why-you-should-eat-oatmeal-
every-day/.

Taylor, Jordyn. "Eating Lots of Healthy Food Will Still Make You Gain
Weight—Here's How." *Tech.Mic.* Mic, 30 December 2015. Web. 26
May 2016. https://mic.com/articles/131516/eating-lots-of-healthy-
food-will-still-make-you-gain-weight-here-s-how#.F0q6hQEWe.

Warner, Jennifer. "30 Minutes of Daily Exercise Enough to Shed Pounds."
WebMD. WebMD, LLC, 24 August 2012. Web. 28 May 2016.
http://www.webmd.com/fitness-exercise/20120824/30-minutes-daily-
exercise-shed-pounds.

"Weight loss: Strategies for success." *Mayo Clinic.* Mayo Foundation for
Medical Education and Research, n.d. Web. 26 March 2016.
http://www.mayoclinic.org/healthy-lifestyle/weight-loss/in-
depth/weight-loss/art-20047752.

"What it Takes to Lose Weight." *Family Doctor.org.* American Academy of
Family Physicians, March 2016. Web. 27 May 2016.
http://familydoctor.org/familydoctor/en/prevention-wellness/food-

nutrition/weight-loss/what-it-takes-to-lose-weight.html.

Whitbread, Daisy. "37 Beans and Legumes with the Most Protein." *HealthAliciousNess.com*. Healthaliciousness.com, n.d. Web. 7 November 2015. http://www.healthaliciousness.com/articles/beans-legumes-highest-protein.php.

Youdim, Adrienne. "Carbohydrates, Proteins, and Fats." *Merck Manual Consumer Version*. Merck Sharp & Dohme Corp., n.d. Web. 18 April 2016. https://www.merckmanuals.com/home/disorders-of-nutrition/overview-of-nutrition/carbohydrates,-proteins,-and-fats.

Younger, Kath. "What Is Real Food?" *Kath Eats Real Food*. N.p., 4 September 2013. Web. 26 May 2016. http://www.katheats.com/what-is-real-food.

Zelman, Kathleen M. "Lose Weight Fast: How to Do It Safely." *WebMD*. WebMD, LLC, n.d. Web. 18 April 2016.

DIET-FREE ME
FREE COMPANION RESOURCES

Some chapters in this book include links to helpful materials intended to help you with your journey of embracing a healthy lifestyle diet-free.

Although the choice is yours of whether or not you care to access that information, I highly recommend you access the information I have created for you at the following website:

pamelaburke.com/dietfreeme-resources

The information you will have access to is free. Who doesn't like FREE?!

The resources include downloadable worksheets, cheat sheets, and other useful content to assist you on your journey to embracing a healthy lifestyle diet-free.

Overt time I will continue to add content to this area, therefore be sure to visit the web address below to get your free instant access now.

Thanks and enjoy!

Visit the following link to get free access to your Diet-Free Me bonus materials now:

pamelaburke.com/dietfreeme-resources

ACKNOWLEDGEMENTS

It took me many years to learn this, but there is not much we can accomplish all by ourselves. This is where I get to acknowledge those who helped me make this book become a reality.

I start with the best part, only second to waking up every day—Kelly. Kelly, when I set out on the journey to lose weight, you supported me. When I decided to start a blog, you supported me. When I decided to become a speaker, you supported me. When I decided to write a book, you supported me. You rightfully worried if I was spreading myself too thin, but there you were, eating healthy with me, exercising with me, editing blog posts for me, and sharing ideas for this book with me. Thank you for being everything for me.

My parents might knock me upside the head for failing to mention the one who makes all things possible—The Good Lord above. Thank you, God. It was out of my greatest pain, self-doubts, and lack of a sense of belonging that you touched me, opening up my mind to my ability to create opportunities. It is out of this that you taught me, guided me, and helped me get out of my way to be able to provide this book, this guide, to help the lives of others. One of the greatest gifts you have given me is to be there for others.

Shout out to my personal trainer, Gail Williams of Simply Fitness. Even as I write this, I can hear you saying, "If I'm not challenging you, I am not changing you." Thank you for constantly reminding me that challenge is a good thing. Any time a self-doubting thought crept into my thoughts about my ability to pull off writing a book, I knew I was being challenged, and each time I kept going, I knew I was changing. I was becoming mentally stronger in my belief that I could do this. Now it is done.

Many people, some of whom I do not know personally, helped in constructing the title for this book. There was one person in particular, however, who let it be known that she was in no way feeling my original ideas. Dana Bryant, you pushed me, girl. I am not sure what the subtitle would have been without you.

To the wonderful women like the ones who read the book early and who are fighting each day because your struggle is real, you have been a blessing to me. Thank You for allowing me to share your truth.

Cristina Olds. Girl, I am sure I got to be a pain in your butt by not knowing what in the world I wanted for the cover of this book. Thank you for being a good sport and for consulting me on what and what not to do.

I have already mentioned I was completely lost when it came to the cover design for the book. I was so torn on what to do that I chose two illustrators for the cover, Faye Saavedra and Anandhito Galih Respati. Ultimately it was Anandhito's design that made the cover, but the decision was not easy. Thank You both.

When you are doing something for the first time it is wise to go to someone who understands the process. Heidi Sutherlin is who helped me through that process. Thank You for finalizing the book cover, formatting the book, and creating my print copy.

Holly Reid, my ATL GA connection. When I speak of God reaching down and touching me, I think of the day I received your email asking me to be your Self-Publishing School (aka SPS) accountability partner. Until you came along, all I was doing was thinking about the book. You came in asking me when I was going to do what when. You got my butt in gear and now I am here.

Jen Henderson. I reached out and you quickly responded. You came through for me. Your promptness, direction, and beautiful nature were calming at a time when I needed it. I appreciate you more than words can say.

Chandler Bolt, the founder of Self-Publishing School, the SPS coaches and its community, wow—what an amazing group of people. The tips and advice you shared so freely, openly, and honestly, were immense help in my writing, completing, publishing, and launching *Diet-Free Me* .

The thought of writing this book would not have happened if not for the people who repeatedly asked me how I lost weight. You all provided my purpose. – Thank You.

ABOUT CAN. WILL. DONE! THE BLOG

canwilldone.com

Can. Will. DONE! is a blog where I share my personal struggles with limiting beliefs and behaviors such as, but surely not limited to, perfectionism, self-doubt, and fear. I also share my weight-loss journey. As I struggled to get healthy and fit again, I realized there was a connection between the battle of the bulge and those already mentioned limiting behaviors.

Can. Will. DONE! is about the myriad of limiting behaviors that not just I but we impose upon ourselves. At its core, Can. Will. DONE! is framed around self-improvement and continuous growth, because bettering ourselves is completely in our hands—it is something we can control.

Each Thursday, subscribers to the blog receive an email on the topic of self-improvement, embracing a healthy lifestyle, or a combination of the two. Each month, these same subscribers receive an inspiration email. I discuss occurrences that I have experienced or witnessed and share them with my readers as a way to encourage and inspire them to live beyond the limitations they have set for themselves.

ABOUT PAMELA BURKE THE SPEAKER

pamelaburke.com

Change Your Mind; Change Your Body

Thin a majority of my life, I gained fifty pounds in my early thirties before taking action to lose the weight. I vowed I would not allow myself to face that type of hurdle again. A decade later, I was mentally broken as the result of gaining one hundred pounds.

After going through and succeeding with the challenge of losing those hundred pounds, I now spend my time sharing and inspiring others with my message of what it takes to start the process of transforming your body and mind for life.

Opportunity Knocks

Experiencing unfavorable life circumstances and situations or witnessing someone else's successes gets inside our heads, leading to thoughts of self-doubt, uncertainty, and life-deflating language, such as "I can't" or "I give up." These thoughts make us believe that our opportunities are limited.

Having changed my life by choosing to live and think differently, I captivate audiences with my empowering message about the formula I use to live life choosing to have a can-do attitude and let audiences know how to create opportunities and understand that we are only limited by our thoughts.

The Missing Message

Having worked in corporate America for nearly a quarter of a century, I recognized late in my career that the directive given to me growing up—"Get good grades so you can go to and graduate from college. Get a job. Work hard."—did not properly prepare me for my working future.

Having a passion for education, for young people who lack exposure and experiences, and for being accountable for your own future, I share lessons I wish I had learned at their age.

ABOUT PAMELA BURKE THE AUTHOR

Pamela Burke is the creator of Can. Will. DONE!—a website dedicated to helping people change their mind, attitude, way of life, and body. Pamela strives to get people to live a can-do attitude in every area of their lives, thus allowing them to change their self-doubts, fears, circumstances, and struggles into positive opportunities. Like with this book, on the website, Pamela also shares advice on how to maintain a healthy lifestyle.

Pamela is also a speaker. She speaks on topics such as creating opportunities, changing mindsets, and living a healthy lifestyle, and to parents and students about the messages they are missing related to attending college.

In addition to speaking to young people about college and education, she also serves as a mentor and provides scholarships to college students.

For the record, Pamela does all of the above work on the side. She has worked in corporate America for twenty-five years, as of the time of this writing. She serves as a co-lead for one of her employer's affinity groups. Always willing to sit on a panel or speak on creating opportunities with work colleagues, she has been graced with the unofficial title of "Good Corporate Citizen." Her daily functions also include helping others, but by way of helping technically with devising more efficient processes and providing data solutions.

Pamela resides in Central New Jersey, where she was born and raised, with the love her life, Kelly.